The
Acid
Alkaline
Diet

for
Optimum Health

The
Acid -
Alkaline
Diet
for
Optimum Health

Restore Your Health by Creating
Balance in Your Diet

CHRISTOPHER VASEY, N.D.

Translated by Jon Graham

Healing Arts Press
Rochester, Vermont

Healing Arts Press
One Park Street
Rochester, Vermont 05767
www.InnerTraditions.com

Healing Arts Press is a division of Inner Traditions International

Note to the reader: This book is intended as an informational guide. The remedies, approaches, and techniques described herein are meant to supplement, and not to be a substitute for, professional medical care or treatment. They should not be used to treat a serious ailment without prior consultation with a qualified health care professional.

Library of Congress Cataloging-in-Publication Data
Vasey, Christopher
  [Gérez votre équilibre acido-basique. English]
  The acid-alkaline diet for optimum health : restore your health by creating balance in your diet / Christopher Vasey ; translated by Jon Graham. – 1st U.S. ed.
     p. cm.
  ISBN 0-89281-099-8 (pbk.)
  1. Diet therapy. 2. Acid-base imbalances—Diet therapy. 3. Acid-base imbalances—Nutritional aspects. 4. Nutritionally induced diseases. I. Title.
  RM216.V36513 2004
  615.8'54—dc22

                                                                2003019921

Printed and bound in Canada at Transcontinental

10 9 8 7 6 5 4

Text design and layout by Priscilla Baker
This book was typeset in Sabon with Avenir as a display typeface

Contents

Introduction

⨍

The importance of the body's acid–alkaline balance to overall health is being recognized by an increasing number of patients and therapists. In my book *L'équilibre acido-basique* (Geneva: Editions Jouvence, 1991), I explained what this balance is and how to correct it when it is lost in order to restore good health.

Experience has shown the need for a more detailed examination of certain points to make this corrective therapy easier to implement for the reader, including how to interpret urine pH measurements, choose corrective foods, create alkaline menus, decide dosages for alkaline supplements, and so forth.

The purpose of *The Acid–Alkaline Balance Diet for Optimal Health* is to shed new light where needed. In this respect it is an eminently practical book. While it will stand perfectly well on its own, it also makes the ideal complement to *L'équilibre acido-basique*.

This book consists of three parts, each corresponding to one of the major questions about acid–alkaline balance.

1. How do I know if I have an acid problem?
Following a brief definition of the acidity problem, part one explains what tests are available, how to perform them, and, most importantly, how to interpret them.

2. How do I lower acidity through diet?
Diet plays a fundamental role in acid–alkaline balance. Part two provides detailed lists of foods that are alkalizing, foods that are acidifying, and foods that are acid; a classification of foods according to their acidifying properties; guidelines for a balanced diet; an analysis of currently popular but acidifying meals; and numerous suggestions for alkaline-based menus.

3. How do I neutralize and eliminate acids?
Treatments using alkaline supplements—which are often applied incorrectly—are explained in part three in detail: dosages, how long a treatment should last, how to monitor the effectiveness of a supplement, what products are available, and so forth. Also explained is how to drain acids from the body and rejuvenate it with alkaline energy-boosters.

By following the guidelines offered in this book, readers affected by acid problems will be working actively toward the recovery of their good health. I wish you every success.

———

Note: The fresh cheese called for in this book can be any of a large number of cheeses that have not been ripened and thus are intended for immediate consumption. American cottage cheese is on this list, as are ricotta, mozzarella, quark, fromage blanc, neufchâtel, and queso blanco. Especially prevalent in the recommendations in this book is fromage blanc for its spreadability; its consistency is also good for mixing with fruits and preserves. Fromage blanc is now available in many health food stores and supermarkets. Good substitutes for fromage blanc are fresh goat cheese, neufchâtel, and soft cream cheese, preferably the low-fat variety.

Cheeses and dairy foods that have a higher whey content will become more acidic as they age—this is why cottage cheese can be found listed as both an alkaline and an acid food. Generally the firmer large-curd cottage cheese will be more alkaline. Consumers should also be aware of the expiration date on the container, as the acidity of cottage cheese increases with age.

Part One

DEFINING ACIDITY

1

What Is Acid–Alkaline Balance?

The substances the body uses for building and functioning are quite numerous: there are approximately twenty amino acids, several dozen sugars and fatty acids, approximately forty vitamins, and one hundred or so minerals and trace elements. Each of these substances plays one or several specific roles in the body.

Despite the extreme diversity of these substances, it is possible to classify them in two major groups: basic (or alkaline) substances and acid substances. These two different groups of substances have opposing but complementary characteristics. To be healthy, the body needs both. When alkalines and acids are present in equal quantities, the acid–alkaline balance is achieved.

Many organic balances are necessary for good health: those between activity and rest, inhalation and exhalation, venous and arterial blood, energy intake and expenditure, and the production and elimination of toxins. Just as it is detrimental to disturb any one of these balances—for example, to eat more than the body needs or not rest enough to make up for daily activity—an excess of either acid or alkaline substances is very harmful to health.

WHAT IS AN ACID?

If you have ever bitten into a lemon or eaten rhubarb you know the most obvious characteristic of an acid: its taste. But acidic foods also stimulate salivation to dilute the acid, which brings out another property of acids—their harsh, even corrosive, nature.

We take advantage of this latter property in everyday life in many ways. Vinegar dissolves the calcium deposits that can form in pots and sinks, and some of today's cleaning products partially owe their cleansing qualities to the acids they contain. The corrosive nature of acids is also demonstrated by the well-known experiment of soaking a piece of meat or a coin in a cola-based beverage. After several days the meat will have dissolved totally and the surface of the coin will be scarred and pitted.

Chemically, acids are defined as substances that release hydrogen ions when dissolved in water. Some acids give off more hydrogen ions than others. Rhubarb and lemons, for example, are much more acidic than strawberries or tomatoes, which are also acidic foods.

Taste is not an infallible means for determining that a food is acidic, because acids can be partially neutralized and their taste obscured by the presence of other substances. Meat and cereal grains are not acidic to the taste, but they are very acidifying foods.

The degree of acidity of a substance is measured by determining its pH (see "How Acidity Is Measured," p. 7). It is also possible to identify a food as acidic by analyzing its mineral content. In fact, minerals can be divided into the same two basic groups: acidic and alkaline. The principal acidic minerals are sulfur, chlorine, phosphorus, fluoride, iodine, and silicon.

When a substance contains more acidic than alkaline minerals it is said to be acidic. Accordingly, mineral waters, which contain both types of mineral, are said to be alkaline when alkaline minerals such as calcium and magnesium predominate and acidic when sulfur, chlorine, or carbon dioxide prevail. A food rich in phosphorus—hazelnuts, for example— is more acidic than one that contains less phosphorus, like almonds.

WHAT IS AN ALKALINE?

Unlike acidic substances, alkaline substances in solution with water give up few or no hydrogen ions. The fewer hydrogen ions they release the less acidic they are—or, in other words, the more alkaline.

Also unlike acids, alkaline elements have no corrosive properties. They are "gentle" substances. Whereas lemon juice causes a sharp burning sensation if applied to a cut, milk does not. Alkaline substances can counter problems caused by acids. Potato juice, for example, soothes the pains of an acid stomach, and milk in large quantities can be an effective method of neutralizing the corrosiveness of acidic poisons swallowed by accident.

Alkaline foods have little or no acidic taste. In the most-alkaline foods, such as bananas, almonds, and fresh milk, not even the slightest trace of an acidic taste can be detected.

Alkaline minerals include calcium, sodium, magnesium,

cobalt, and copper. The body contains more calcium than any other mineral, more than two pounds on average, most of which is concentrated in the skeleton.

As with acids, flavor is not a sufficient criterion for determining whether a food is alkaline. Certain foods—for example, bread and white sugar—are not at all acidic to the taste, but they are not alkaline foods. The acids these foods contain are freed in the course of their digestion and utilization by the body.

HOW ACIDITY IS MEASURED

As the difference between an acid and an alkaline is based more or less on their ability to free hydrogen ions, the unit that measures the degree of acidity or alkalinity of a substance is shorthand for the substance's potential (p) for freeing hydrogen (H) ions, or pH.

The pH measuring scale goes from 0 to 14. The number 7 indicates the ideal balance between acids and alkaline substances and is known as a neutral pH. The greater potential a substance has for freeing hydrogen ions, the smaller is its pH number. The acidity range is from 6 to 0, zero indicating a state of absolute acidity. Conversely, a more alkaline pH is indicated by a higher figure, from 8 to 14, the last figure representing a state of total alkalinity (meaning a state in which no hydrogen ions are freed).

The pH scale

Note that on the pH measurement scale, the *greater* the degree of acidity, the *lower* the pH reading.

It is important to know that the transition from one figure to the next on this scale of measurement is not arithmetical but logarithmic, meaning that the values separating each unit are not of equal value along the scale but increase in proportion to their distance from the midway point of an even balance between acidity and alkalinity. The values are multiplied by 10 at each unit (see diagram, "The pH scale," p. 7). In other words, if the concentration of hydrogen ions is 10 at a pH reading of 6 it will be 100 at a pH reading of 5; 1,000 at a pH reading of 4; 10,000 at a pH reading of 3; and so on. The gap between a pH of 6 and a pH of 5, for example, is not equal to the gap between a pH of 5 and a pH of 4; a gap of 90 in the first case becomes a gap of 900 in the second.

This means that the degree of acidity is much greater than one might think from the progression of the figures. Consequently, when urinary pH falls, for example, from 6 to 5, it is registering a much greater amount of acidification than that indicated by a decrease from 7 to 6.

The pH of different substances can be measured with a special reactive paper known as litmus paper. When put into contact with a dilution of the substance to be tested, the paper changes color to a degree that corresponds to the degree of acidity or alkalinity of that substance.

DIFFERENCE BETWEEN STRONG AND WEAK ACIDS

In addition to the degree of acidity as measured by the pH scale, acids can be characterized as either strong or weak. In

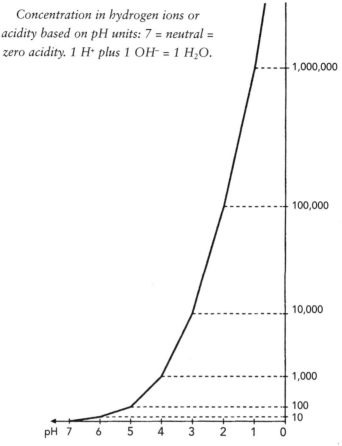

Concentration in hydrogen ions or acidity based on pH units: 7 = neutral = zero acidity. 1 H⁺ plus 1 OH⁻ = 1 H₂O.

From the book *Terrain acidifié* by Jacques Fontaine (Geneva: Editions Jouvence, 1990).

fact, acids are rarely encountered in a free or isolated state; they are most often combined with an alkaline element. When the alkaline combined with the acid is strong (chemically speaking), the acid is of little consequence in the combination. The acid is called weak, as it is easy for the body to reject it. When the alkaline element is weak, however, the acid content is of much greater consequence. It is stable and mixes poorly with other elements, and it is referred to as strong.

Physiologically, strong acids—precisely because of their stability and resistance to combining—are much more difficult to neutralize and eliminate from the body than weak acids.

Strong acids come primarily from animal proteins. They chiefly consist of uric, sulfuric, and phosphoric acids. Their elimination from the body requires significant neutralization, a task performed by the liver as well as the normal elimination work of the kidneys. Because the kidneys can only eliminate a fixed amount of strong acids on a daily basis, however, any excess is stored in the tissues. Consequently, it is important to monitor the consumption of animal proteins.

Weak acids are primarily of plant origin (carbohydrates and vegetable proteins), except for those coming from yogurt and whey, which are of animal origin. Weak acids include citric, oxalic, pyruvic, and acetylsalicylic acids. Weak acids are also called volatile acids,* because once they have been oxidized they are eliminated by the lungs in the form of vapors and gases, both as breath moisture and as carbon dioxide (CO_2). Their elimination is relatively easy, and there are no limits on the quantity that can be expelled from the body by the kidneys, unlike nonvolatile strong acids. When the body needs to increase the elimination of volatile acids it does so simply by increasing the rate of respiration. The amount of volatile acids that can be eliminated is limited only by how fast and how deeply a person is able to breathe.

---

*Volatile acids are primarily regulated by respiratory function, as opposed to fixed acids, which can only be regulated by the kidneys and eliminated from the body in fluid form.

pH AND HEALTH

The body functions at its best when the pH of its internal bio-chemical environment, measured as a whole, is equal to 7.39, meaning slightly alkaline. The normal range of this optimum pH is very small, from a slightly more acidic reading of 7.36 to a more alkaline reading of 7.42. A reading of anything higher or lower than these figures indicates acidosis (from 7.36 to 7) or alkalosis (7.42 to 7.8). If these limits are exceeded, the body can no longer function, and death results.

Fatal acidosis to fatal alkalosis

The zone of optimal health extends only from pH 7.36 to pH 7.42; illness will accompany any incidence of acidosis or alkalosis. Of these two, acidosis is by far the most common—more than half the population suffers from this condition. This is what we concentrate on in the remainder of the book.

The pH of the body's organic fluids and tissues varies from one part of the body to another. When we say the ideal pH of the body is 7.39, this refers primarily to the pH of the blood, and to a lesser extent that of the body's internal environment, meaning all organic fluids such as lymph and extra- and intracellular serums (fluids surrounding or within the cells). Blood is indeed "a very particular sap" (Goethe) whose pH must remain extremely stable to maintain the life of the physical organism. Even the slightest change of blood pH is rapidly corrected by the body, which restores it to the ideal measurement of 7.39. When the body is unable to perform this task physical and mental disorders quickly appear.

The pH of the internal environment, the basic "ground" biochemical terrain, can tolerate more significant changes than that of the blood, but the pH of the internal environment should never go beyond 7.36 or 7.42 if good health is to be maintained.

Many individual organs and organic fluids, however, have a pH that is normally far above or below this ideal pH. The pH of urine, for example, may be 6, or even as low as 5 or 4.5. This is possible because urine is regularly eliminated and thus does not remain in the body for long. Areas of the body that are essentially acid include the small intestine (pH 6), the outer layers of the skin (pH 5.2), and the gastric region (pH 2). Others, in contrast, are quite alkaline: the inner layers of the skin (pH 7.35), the pancreatic juices (from pH 7.5 to 8.8), and the large intestine (pH 8).

These different values are all normal and correspond to precise needs of the body. For example, the extremely acidic nature of the gastric region is indispensable for protein digestion, and the high acidity of the skin helps it destroy microbes before they can enter the body.

So restoring the acid–alkaline balance does not mean bringing the gastric region's pH 2 up to pH 7—that would cause serious digestive problems—but rather restoring the pH of the basic internal biochemical terrain. The acidification of the internal terrain is in fact the source of all health troubles caused by acidity.

HOW THE BODY DEFENDS ITSELF
AGAINST ACIDIFICATION

Whenever there is an imbalance between acid and alkaline substances, whether in the body's entire system or a particular organ, the body is forced to react in self-defense. It has two means at its disposal to take action: to reduce the amount of the excessive substance by eliminating it from the body; and to partially neutralize the substance by forming neutral salts with the help of elements whose properties are the opposite of those causing the problem.

Let's examine the first of these solutions more closely.

The task of getting rid of excess acid in the body falls to the organs responsible for elimination: the lungs and kidneys.

The most rapid means for getting rid of a sudden intake of acids is via the respiratory system. By oxidizing acids the lungs release them with each breath in the form of carbon dioxide and breath moisture. This is a fairly easy solution, as it simply requires increasing the volume and rate of the breath to intensify the pace of elimination and adapt it to the body's immediate physical needs.

Unfortunately, this method is capable of dealing only with weak acids. Fixed acids, which are nonvolatile and cannot be exhaled as a gas by the lungs, can be eliminated through the kidneys only in a solid form. Uric, sulfuric, and similar acids must therefore be filtered out of the bloodstream by the kidneys and sent out of the body diluted in the urine. The kidneys, unlike the lungs, cannot adapt their elimination potential in accord with the needs of the body. Even working at maximum capacity, the kidneys cannot eliminate more than a certain daily fixed amount.

The accumulation of excess acid in the body's internal environment would be irremediable if there was not another exit available: the skin, specifically the sweat glands. Often the skin is overlooked as a means of elimination, but it is very useful for the disposal of acids.

Distributed over the entire surface of the skin, the sweat glands—of which there are more than 2 million—can expel strong acids because they work similarly to the kidneys and eliminate the same kind of wastes. Strong acids can be flushed from the body diluted in sweat, although in lesser quantities than in urine, as the body loses less than a quart of sweat a day compared to about one and a half quarts of urine. Furthermore, sweat carries a much smaller amount of toxins than does urine.

THE BUFFER SYSTEM

Acids and alkaline substances possess opposing characteristics. When they combine, their respective properties cancel each other out. This process is similar to what occurs whenever two opposites are brought together. If hot and cold, or black and white, are blended, their respective properties cancel each other out, and the result is a temperature that is neither hot nor cold but warm, or a color that is neither black nor white but gray.

The combination of an acid and an alkaline is designated in chemistry as a neutral salt. It is neutral because it possesses neither acidic nor alkaline properties.

1 acid + 1 alkaline = 1 neutral salt

A neutral salt no longer influences the solution it is in, such as blood or cellular serums. Neutralization of excess acids restores the acid–alkaline balance to the ideal pH of the internal environment, 7.39, which is itself almost neutral.

The alkaline substances the body uses to neutralize or buffer strong acids, or the sudden intake of a massive amount of weak acids, can be found throughout the body, not just in the blood. Alkaline substances in the bloodstream are utilized, but because blood pH can fluctuate only slightly, they are only minimally drawn upon. Instead the body makes use of alkaline elements found in less important parts of the body, such the tissues of the internal organs.

When this defense system is used only occasionally, the alkaline elements thus lost are easily replaced by the alkaline minerals found in food, and the tissues suffer no ill effects from making what amounts to a loan of their alkaline components. Problems occur, however, when the tissues are forced to relinquish their alkaline elements on a regular basis, every day or even several times a day. In this case the body's alkaline reserves inevitably gradually diminish. The word *reserves*, it should be noted, is something of a misnomer; these alkaline substances have not been set aside by the body for the express purpose of dealing with excess acid. These minerals are components of the tissues themselves and fulfill a very precise role in that regard.

Repeated withdrawals therefore create a shortage of alkaline minerals in these organic tissues. The critical mineral loss becomes even more pronounced when the plundering is intense and prolonged. Modern lifestyle and diet encourage such exploitation of the body's buffer system. It is the source of a host of troubles and diseases, as well as the general sense of malaise suffered by many in our contemporary civilization.

HOW ACIDIFICATION MAKES THE BODY SICK

When its internal environment becomes acidified, the body can fall ill in three different ways.

The first is connected to the activity of enzymes. Enzymes are the "worker drones" behind all the biochemical transformations that take place in the body and on which the proper functioning of the organs depend. Enzymes can perform their task correctly only in an environment with a clearly defined pH; otherwise their activity can be disrupted or even cease completely. When their activity is merely slowed down, illness appears. If there is a complete interruption the body can no longer function, and death results. Before this extreme stage is reached, different ailments set in as an increasing number of enzymes find their world disturbed by the acidification of the internal environment.

The second way the body becomes ill is due to the harsh, corrosive nature of acids present in excess amounts within the tissues. Before they are neutralized by alkaline substances, the acids irritate the organ with which they come in contact. Inflammation, sometimes quite painful, results, as well as lesions or hardening of the tissues. This primarily affects the organs charged with the elimination of strong acids, such as the skin and kidneys. Many cases of eczema, hives, itching, and red patches on the skin are due to the irritation caused by excessively acidic sweat. The most susceptible regions are those where sweat has a tendency to collect: in the armpits, behind the knees, under the wristwatch band, or, in babies, under the diaper. When the urine is overloaded with acid urination is painful and the urinary tract "burns," becoming inflamed (urethritis) or infected (cystitis).

Ailments triggered by harsh acid that are invisible to the outsider but are keenly felt by the victims include pains in the joints (arthritis), nerves (neuritis), and intestines (enteritis, colitis, and burning sensations in the anus).

The fragile state of the tissues resulting from the invasive presence of acid makes them vulnerable to microbial or viral infection as well. Lesions of the mucous membranes—such as in the respiratory system—allow easier penetration and multiplication by microbes in the tissues. This is aggravated by the fact that the immune system's effectiveness can also be impaired by acid activity, which lowers the production and strength of the white blood cells responsible for attacking microbes.

The third cause of suffering from excess acid is loss of minerals, since the body gives up alkaline minerals to neutralize acids. This demineralization can be quite significant and can affect any organ because alkaline minerals are stored in all the body's tissues.

The best-known consequences of demineralization are problems affecting the skeleton and teeth. Bones lose their calcium, and along with it their resistance and flexibility, to the point where they break far too easily (for example, spontaneous hip fractures), lose their density (osteoporosis), become inflamed at the joints (rheumatism), wear away the intervertebral disks (sciatica), and so forth. Teeth can also become more brittle because of mineral loss. They can chip, become oversensitive to hot and cold foods, or become more susceptible to cavities.

The brittleness caused by demineralization also weakens hair, which loses its shine and resilience and starts falling out in greater quantity. Fingernails split and break under the slightest impact; skin dries and cracks or wrinkles; the gums become deformed and oversensitive and bleed easily.

ILLNESSES CAUSED BY ACIDIFICATION

Acidification engenders many afflictions that manifest in various ways. An individual suffering from excessive acid will not contract them all, only those that take advantage of the person's specific physiological weaknesses. Weak points are determined by temperament, heredity, accidents, lifestyle, and sometimes profession. With some people it is primarily the skin or respiratory system that is afflicted; with others it is the nerves or teeth, the gums, the eyes, or the spinal column.

Besides the illnesses listed above, acidification of the internal environment leads to great fatigue, even in the absence of any physical or mental effort. Generally the person afflicted no longer has any drive or enthusiasm, tires quickly, and takes a long time to recover from exertion. The individual tends to be touchy and irritable, to worry too much, and to sleep poorly, and may even become depressed. The noxious effect of acids on the nerves is easily explained: minerals like magnesium, calcium, and potassium that the nervous system needs to function properly are precisely the alkaline minerals the body takes away to neutralize acids.

Individuals suffering from acidification often are sensitive to the cold, have low blood pressure, and are subject to episodes of low blood sugar. All the functions of the endocrine glands tend to slow down, except for those of the thyroid gland, which become hyperactive. The immune system is weakened as well, and recurring infections of the respiratory tract (colds, laryngitis, flu, bronchitis) or urinary tract (cystitis) appear with distressing frequency due to the combination of low immune response and the ease with which microbes can penetrate the body through tiny lesions in the mucous membranes of the respiratory and urinary tracts.

A surprising number and variety of physical problems and diseases can be caused by acidity. Indeed, a triple action can prompt their appearance: enzymatic disturbances, aggressive activity by acids, and demineralization are three factors capable of striking any organic tissue.

Of course, such problems are not always caused solely by acids. Bleeding gums, for example, can be the result of poor dental hygiene or a lack of vitamin C. But a person suffering from excessive acidity is often simultaneously or successively stricken by several of these afflictions. As varied as the conditions may appear, however, such a person's troubles can all be remedied by one treatment: the deacidification of the internal environment.

ACIDOSIS: A WIDESPREAD PROBLEM

Today the vast majority of the populace in Western (industrialized) nations suffers from problems caused by acidification, because both modern lifestyle and diet promote acidification of the body's internal environment.

In general, the current standard diet is primarily composed of acidic or acidifying elements (proteins, cereals, sugars). Alkaline foods such as vegetables are eaten in much smaller quantities; their alkaline content is insufficient to neutralize surplus acids. Furthermore, the consumption of stimulants like tobacco, coffee, tea, and alcohol—every one of which has an extremely acidifying effect on the body—has grown to enormous proportions.

Stress, nervous tension, noise, shortage of time, and other pressures are facts of life today and contribute to increasing the body's acidification through the physiological disturbances they create.

Physical exercise—which can play an important role in maintaining acid–alkaline balance—is more often than not either insufficient or excessive. In both cases, acidification of the body's internal environment is the result.

Of all the factors causing acidification, the most important is unquestionably food. The majority of acidosis sufferers can be treated simply by significantly reducing their consumption of acids and increasing their consumption of alkaline foods.

There is a special category of individuals, however, who are sick not only because of inadequate lifestyle and an excessive intake of acids. They also suffer from a metabolic weakness that is particularly susceptible to acids.

Some illnesses arise because a person's body is unable to properly metabolize a particular nutrient. Partially or completely unmetabolized nutrients stagnate in the body, causing it to fall ill either through their own toxic effects or by disrupting the body's functioning. In diabetes, for example, the substance that is poorly metabolized is sugar; in rheumatism it is proteins; in obesity it is fat; in celiac disease it is gluten; and in water retention it is salt. These are just a few of the many substances, acids among them, that the body may have trouble metabolizing.

Difficulty metabolizing acids primarily involves weak acids. Weak acids are normally quite easy to oxidize, and their elimination through the lungs in the form of carbon dioxide or breath moisture makes the strong alkaline substances with which they had been combined available for the body's use. As a rule, foods rich in weak acids, such as fruits, whey, yogurt, and vinegar, contribute a large number of alkaline elements to the body. But this is not always true for everyone, specifically that category of people whose metabolisms have trouble oxidizing weak acids.

For such people, acids are poorly oxidized, if at all, and these substances remain in the body without releasing the alkaline substances with which they are combined. In people with this metabolic weakness, foods that would normally contribute a high quota of alkaline substances instead have the effect of acidifying the internal environment. The same food can have an entirely different effect depending on the body of the person who ingests it. This is why some dietitians declare that lemon is an alkalizing food while others claim it is acidifying. Both are correct. The error lies in not determining whether the physical constitution of the person eating that kind of food has an inherent metabolic weakness toward acids.

People afflicted with this metabolic debility must take additional precautions with their diets. It is essential that they carefully regulate the amount of foods they eat that are rich in weak acids (see the list "Acid Foods" in chapter 3, p. 60).

Normally, this group of "acid foods" doesn't figure in the classifications set up to help people maintain their acid–alkaline balance. Foods are generally divided into only two groups: acidifying and alkalizing. Acid foods are usually included in the list of alkalizing foods, since with their weak acids they have an alkalizing effect on most people. But the lack of a third list of acid foods could lead to serious problems for individuals whose metabolic Achilles heel is acids. They could consume large quantities of fruits, vinegar, and so on, confident they were alkalizing their internal environments, whereas in fact they were creating precisely the opposite effect.

HEALING THE PROBLEMS CAUSED BY ACIDIFICATION

The problems caused by acidification should not be treated individually, but as a whole. Because acidification of the internal environment is responsible for so many different symptoms and illnesses, the most effective treatment for these conditions is to reduce or eliminate acidification. This is the surest way to make all the problems it has caused disappear.

Simple treatment of surface symptoms may bring relief, but it provides very little in the way of long-term effects because the fundamental imbalance in the body's internal environment remains unchanged. Treating only the symptoms forces the sufferer to run from one specialist to another, spending the morning at the dermatologist's getting treatment for eczema, then dividing the afternoon between the rheumatologist for painful joints and the dentist for gum problems. In contrast, focusing treatment on the main problem—reversing the acidification of the body's internal environment—goes to work right at the root of these ailments and treats them all.

The treatment plan to counter acidification aims first to reduce the amount of acids the body takes in. This is an indispensable step; as long as large quantities of acids are entering the body, all other measures have only a temporary palliative effect. Diet is adjusted so that alkaline foods and drinks predominate over acid foods. Dietary reform is a simple step, but its effect is considerable. Improved oxidation of acids is obtained by introducing or increasing physical activity (walking, sports). Eliminating the acids already present in the tissues is accelerated by consuming medicinal plants that increase the flow of urine (diuretics) and those that enhance the production of sweat (sudorifics).

An additional measure, which has proven to be indispensable in the majority of cases, is to take alkaline mineral supplements, not only to help the body eliminate the acids ingested during the day but also, and more importantly, to facilitate elimination of the acids lodged in the deep tissues of the body. This is a fundamental step, because the body is extremely reluctant to take acids embedded in the tissues back into the bloodstream where they can be transported to the lungs, kidneys, and skin for elimination. The return of acids to the blood carries a serious risk of dangerously altering its pH. To protect the blood, the body tends to let these acids remain in the tissues. However, a significant introduction of alkaline elements into the body allows the acids to be eliminated, for these alkaline substances act as a buffer and let the acids make their way back to the surface in the form of neutral salts. In this form they can cause no harm to the blood pH.

The various measures that can be taken to deacidify the body's internal environment (explained at length in parts two and three) cause all the acids embedded in the deep tissue to gradually resurface and be eliminated. Over time this cleansing leads to a profound deacidification of the body, which not only treats the sufferer but protects him or her from any reoccurrence of the problems.

2

Detecting
Acidification

How can you tell if you are suffering from acidification? There are several tests that are easy to perform and interpret. The most important is also the most common, the test that measures urinary pH. Most often, however, you need to have the results of this test confirmed by another test.

Although two tests performed in a complementary way are enough for a professional to determine if your internal environment is acidic, it is interesting to perform them all, because each reveals another aspect of your physiology, especially with regard to the elements that come into play to make the body acidic.

TEST 1: ANALYSIS OF URINARY pH

As noted, the test for determining the pH of the urine is simple to perform and gives fairly significant information on the degree of acidification from which you may be suffering. It consists of measuring the pH of the urine with litmus paper, which is a paper specially manufactured to make this kind of measurement.

To maintain good health the body is constantly seeking to get rid of the excess acids that irritate the tissues and deplete them of minerals. One of the principal exits it uses for this purpose is the renal system (kidneys). The normal rate of acid excretion through the kidneys gives urine a pH that falls between 7 and 7.5. By testing the degree of acidity of the urine, you can determine whether your body is rejecting a normal quantity of acids. If the excretion rate is higher than normal, the urinary pH will also be more acid, the sign of an overflow of acids that the body is attempting to get rid of. But this overflow is also an indication that the body is saturated and therefore in an acid state, with all the detriments that this can have on your health.

There is thus a close correspondence between the acid pH of the body's internal environment and that of the urine: urine becomes acidic when the body's internal environment becomes acidic. But the value of this test does not stop there. As we will see later in this section, charting how and when urinary pH is either neutral or alkaline yields other valuable information on the state of the internal environment and the way the body is metabolizing acids.

Necessary Materials

To measure urinary pH, all you need is litmus paper, which can be purchased in drugstores, pharmacies, and some health food stores.

Litmus paper has properties that cause it to change color when it comes in contact with acidic or alkaline substances. The color it changes to when in contact with a substance tells you whether the substance is acid or alkaline. It even indicates the strength of the acidity or alkalinity of a substance because the color change becomes more intense if a substance exhibits an extreme pH.

Litmus paper gets its name from the Scandinavian word for certain mosses and lichens that provide the dye that gives the paper its color. This coloring material turns red in acid solutions and blue in alkaline solutions. The neutral blue-violet dye usually comes from a plant in the Euphorbiacea family, such as the croton, though Mediterranean lichens are also often used.

The different shades of color that the coloring agent adopts allow the degree of a substance's acidity or alkalinity to be measured. Each shade of color corresponds to a precise pH value. The value is not indicated on the litmus paper itself, however, but on a color chart that comes with the paper. This chart includes every shade of color the litmus paper can adopt, with its corresponding pH value next to it.

The most common litmus papers available allow pH measurements between 4.5 and 9 to be taken; others have a narrower range of between 5.2 and 7.4. The clearly visible changes of one shade to the next are provided either in half units, which results in a scale that runs 4.5–5.0–5.5–6.0, and so on; or in measurements from 0.2 to 0.4, for example 5.2–5.5–5.8–6.2, and so on. Both systems are sufficiently precise for testing urinary pH.

A large variety of litmus papers is available. In pharmacies and drugstores you can buy the Neutralit Merck or Ames brands. Several other brands are packaged with alkaline mineral supplements that are sold commercially for the purpose of correcting the pH of the internal environment (for more on these see chapter 6).

The paper is sold in rolls from which pieces can be torn as needed, in small rectangular packets that are precut to the desired size, or even as small rods on which this reactive paper has been glued.

The shades of the colors varies according to manufacturer. Some papers go from yellow to blue, others from yellow to red. The transition from one shade of color to the next is obvious enough on any one of these papers to avoid any possibility of confusion. Some brands offer rods on which three different shades of colors are displayed simultaneously in order to make reading them easier.

How to Proceed

Litmus paper needs to be put in contact with the substance to be tested. The most simple method consists of holding the paper in the flow of urine for one or two seconds, just long enough to moisten it. The acid of the urine reacts with the paper, causing it to change color. The paper is then matched to the indicator scale on the color chart. The figure of the corresponding urinary pH is located right next to the color. Remember that it is neutral at 7; at 6.5 and under it is acid; and at 7.5 and above it is alkaline.

A single measurement is not enough to draw any valid conclusions about the state of the internal environment; pH can vary at different times of the day because of activity, meals, physical effort, stress, and so forth. To be truly representative, the measurements must be taken several times a day for four to five days in succession. You should note the data collected from these readings on a chart (see diagram, "Urinary pH Record," p. 28) to obtain an overall picture of pH over time.

As a rule, the first urination in the morning is not representative of your normal pH because it contains all the acids

filtered by the kidneys that have accumulated overnight. The
first test should therefore be made with the second urination
of the morning. The second test should be made on the urine
before lunch, and the third before the evening meal. It is very
important to take the test before the meal, because the pH
can temporarily vary significantly depending on what beverages and foods you have consumed. Besides these three tests,
you may measure and note urine pH at other times of the day
just as complementary data.

The chart on which the measurements of urine pH are
listed consists of five columns, as shown in the example below.

URINARY pH RECORD

Date	Morning	Noon	Evening	Observations
6.1.03	7	7.5	7	had dinner at a restaurant
6.2.03	5	6.5	6.5	
6.3.03	7	7.5	6	stressful afternoon at work
6.4.03	7	7.5	7	

The first column is for the dates on which you take the
measurements. The three following columns are for the morning, noon, and evening readings (from urinating before the
meal). The fifth column is for recording potentially significant
events that may have influenced the pH value—for example,
an especially large meal or one that differs from your usual
fare, a meal at a restaurant, alcohol consumption, an extra
workload, playing sports, a significant amount of stress, or
other various tensions. Be aware that the effects of events such

as these on urinary pH do not always appear on the same day the events occurred but sometimes on the following day, when one or two pH readings may differ from their norms.

You can easily draw such a chart yourself, but a ready-to-use chart is included in the appendix for you to photocopy so you always have a clean copy for reference.

After a week or two there will be enough data to reveal a predominant pH value for each day, as well as for each segment of the day. Except for variations that are due to changes from your habitual activity or other significant incidents, these values should remain relatively constant over time.

How to Interpret the Results

Readings of urinary pH can have only three possible results: under 7, between 7 and 7.5, and above 7.5. While the interpretation of a pH below 7 is a simple matter, because it always indicates that the individual's internal environment has become acidified, this is not the case with the other two possible readings, which require a small additional analysis.

pH Below 7 (Indicative of an Acid pH)

A pH in this range testifies to acidic urine. Regular readings indicating acidic urine are an unmistakable revelation that the body's internal environment is also acidic. This acidification is more significant if the reading is low. A reading of 6 or 6.5 indicates that there is only a slight degree of acidification, but the internal environment is extremely acidic if the urinary acid gives a reading of 5 or 4.5. Anyone obtaining consistent readings in this latter range is strongly advised to adopt without delay the methods for removing acid from the body discussed in parts two and three of this book.

pH Between 7 and 7.5 (Indicative of a Neutral pH)

This is the normal pH of a person in good health and is what you are aiming for. A reading in this range indicates a good acid–alkaline balance *as long as the first urination of the day is acidic*, reflecting all the accumulated acids eliminated by the body during the night. If the first urine is not acidic it is a sign that acids are remaining in the body because the kidneys are not flushing them out properly. This means the internal environment is acidified even if urinary pH readings taken at other times of the day are neutral. Other tests involving foods and symptoms, discussed later in this chapter, can confirm this.

If your first urination of the day is neutral rather than acidic, you are suffering from acidification and should apply the necessary measures to address this problem, with a particular emphasis on the elimination of acids by the skin and kidneys. In fact, in this case an important piece of the problem resides in the eliminatory weakness of these organs.

pH Above 7.5 (Indicative of an Alkaline pH)

As with a neutral pH, there are subtle issues to be considered in interpreting urine pH readings that are consistently above 7.5. There are three possibilities to consider.

First, the internal environment has a good acid–alkaline balance or is slightly alkaline. Generally speaking, this is the case when the food eaten is particularly alkalizing, as is the case with some vegetarians who eat only small quantities of grains and dairy products. Such a reading may also be found for a person who takes alkaline mineral supplements on a daily basis when the body either does not need them or does not need so much of them.

INTERPRETING URINARY pH READINGS

pH	Urine quality	Internal environment quality	Note	Steps to take
below 7	acid	acid	acidifying lifestyle, or metabolism that has trouble with acids	deacidify the body
between 7 and 7.5	neutral	neutral	good health if first urination of the day is acid	maintain current hygiene
		acid	if first urination of the day is also neutral, metabolic inability to handle acids	deacidify internal environment, stimulate kidneys and skin
over 7.5	alkaline	alkaline	vegetarian diet or excessive use of alkaline mineral supplements	maintain current hygiene but avoid protein deficiency
				reduce intake of alkaline minerals
		acid	metabolic inability to handle acids	deacidify internal environment

These specific situations do not signify an imbalance or disease, but some precautions should be taken. Vegetarians must be careful to avoid deficiencies in their diets, especially of proteins. Those taking alkaline supplements should reduce their intake to a level that makes the pH of the urine neutral. (For more on this topic see chapter 6.)

Second, people who have a urinary pH clearly above 7.5 may be suffering from a glandular problem (adrenal or parathyroid glands) or other specific illnesses. These cases are extremely rare, and the people involved are generally already following a medical treatment plan for the problems caused by this imbalance.

The third possibility is the most likely: the urine is alkaline but the internal environment, paradoxically, is acidic. In this case the alkaline pH of the urine is not due to excessive intake of alkaline elements through diet (which the body attempts to get rid of, just as it does with excess acids), but to disproportionate withdrawal of alkaline substances from the organic tissues to neutralize heavy acidification of the internal environment.

This is common among people whose metabolism has difficulty digesting acids. Because the acids are poorly oxidized, they cannot leave the body through the respiratory system. The kidneys must pick up the slack and do double duty of elimination. Although these are the acids classified as weak, their accumulation is dangerous for the body, which will take extreme efforts to buffer itself against the avalanche of acids confronting it. This levy results in bringing a large quantity of alkaline elements into the urine and thus alkalizing it.

The urine is therefore alkaline not because of a net physiological gain in the quantity of alkaline substances, but because of a massive loss of alkaline elements due to the body's plunder of its reserves. This can easily be confirmed by analyzing the types of conditions a person in this situation suffers from to see whether they are among those caused by acidification. In this case it is extremely important to make the internal environment less acidic despite the alkalinity of the urine.

If the pH readings are not uniform during the course of the day, as in the cases mentioned above, but their variations occur regularly at specific times—for example, the urinary pH is acidic in the evening but neutral the rest of the day (except for the first urination of the morning), or vice versa—this indicates an excess of acidity in the internal environment and signals the necessity for restoring it to a neutral state.

TEST 2: ANALYSIS OF SYMPTOMS

Acid aggression on the tissues and the plundering of the body's reserves of alkaline minerals cause characteristic problems. One of the means used for determining whether a person's internal environment is acidified involves analyzing whether any problems he or she is suffering from currently, as well as those that were present in the past, are characteristic of those that accompany acidification.

The list below starts with the description of general symptoms and continues with ailments classified according to the parts of the body they affect.

If you are suffering from only one or two of the problems cited, your internal environment most likely is not acidified; or, if it is, the other characteristic problems have yet to manifest. To learn more you need to perform a test of urinary pH.

Of course, if you are afflicted with acidification you will not suffer from all the problems on the list. When reading the descriptions of these different problems, you may recognize some as conditions you had in the past and others as those you are currently dealing with. You may also recognize some as conditions to which you are susceptible even though you are not currently suffering from their full-blown versions. For example, you might have a tendency toward dry skin or joint pains without actually having eczema or rheumatism.

OVERALL STATE OF HEALTH

• Lack of energy: constant fatigue, loss of physical tone and psychic drive, decreasing activity, tires easily, difficulty in recovering strength following physical or mental effort, sensation of heaviness in the limbs, frequent and sudden feelings of inability to cope, sudden loss of energy following the consumption of acid foods
• Lower body temperature: sensations of intense and deep inner chills, frequently feels cold
• Weight loss specifically due to the decalcification of the bones
• Tendency to get infections because of decreased effectiveness of the body's defenses

MENTAL CONDITION

• Loss of drive, joy, and enthusiasm
• Sadness, dark thoughts, depressive tendencies
• High irritability
• Nervousness: agitation without cause, hyperactivity, sensitivity to high-pitched noises and often startled by them, easily stressed, difficulty dealing with stress

HEAD

- Very pale face (due to capillary contraction)
- Headaches
- Eyes tear easily and are sensitive (to cold, smoke, etc.)
- Conjunctivitis
- Inflammation of the corneas and eyelids

MOUTH

- Acidic saliva
- Loose teeth
- Inflamed, sensitive gums
- Mouth ulcers
- Cracks at the corners of the lips
- Irritation of throat and tonsils that leads to recurring infections

TEETH

- Teeth are sensitive to hot, cold, or acidic foods
- Dental cavities
- Teeth have a tendency to crack or chip
- Pain in the nerves of the teeth
- Acids attack teeth externally (through acidic foods and saliva) and internally (acidic blood)

STOMACH

- Excess stomach acid
- Acid regurgitation
- Stomach pains and spasms
- Gastritis
- Ulcers

INTESTINES

- Diarrhea attacks that expel acids
- Rectal burning sensation
- Predisposition to intestinal inflammation (enteritis, colitis)
- Discoloration of the stools from liver exhaustion
- Anal fistula and cracking
- Tendency to diarrhea
- Cramps and abdominal pains

KIDNEYS AND BLADDER

- Acidic urine
- Burning and irritation in the bladder or urethra
- Excessive urination due to renal irritation
- Kidney and bladder stones

RESPIRATORY SYSTEM

- Runny nose
- Extreme sensitivity of respiratory tract to cold
- Prone to chills
- Frequent colds and bronchitis
- Sinusitis
- Angina (chest pain)
- Laryngitis
- Enlarged tonsils
- Adenoids
- Allergic tendencies
- Coughs and sore throats caused by irritation

SKIN

- Acidic sweat
- Dry skin

- Skin tends to be red and irritated in regions where there are heavy concentrations of sweat (knees, elbows, underarms, around the waist, under the band of a wristwatch or under rings that tarnish), or around openings (eyes, mouth, anus, vulva)
- Skin splits and cracks between fingers and at fingernails
- Fungal diseases
- Hives
- Itches
- Pimples
- Variety of types of eczema, but most commonly dry eczema

NAILS AND HAIR

- Nails are thin and split and break easily
- White streaks or spots on nails
- Hair looks dull, has split ends, and falls out in noticeable quantities

MUSCLES

- Leg cramps and spasms
- Stiff neck and a general sensation of aching all over
- Muscles of the nape of the neck and shoulders tend to be hard and painful

SKELETAL AND JOINT SYSTEM

- Mineral and calcium depletion of the skeleton
- Osteoporosis
- Rickets
- Tendency toward fractures (hip bone), which are slow to heal
- Joints crack

- Joint hyperlaxity
- Locking vertebrae
- Rheumatism
- Arthritis
- Sciatica
- Slipped vertebrae
- Herniated disks
- Inflammation and hardening of the ligaments
- Tendinitis
- Migrant joint pains
- Lumbar pains
- Gout

CIRCULATORY SYSTEM

- Low blood pressure
- Poor circulation
- Tendency to feel cold
- Tendency to suffer from anemia and internal bleeding
- Chilblains
- Rapid heartbeat

ENDOCRINE GLANDS

- Exhaustion and poor function of glands generally, except for the thyroid, which tends to be overactive

GENITAL ORGANS

- Inflammation of the genital tract by acids and infections (itching, swelling, inflammation of the uterus or vulva)
- Vaginal discharge

NERVOUS SYSTEM

- Acute sensitivity to pain anywhere in the body
- Tenacious or migrant nerve pain
- Insomnia
- Nevritis (tennis elbow)

TEST 3: FOOD ANALYSIS

Acids do not appear spontaneously in the organism but have a very specific source: they come from food intake—everything we eat, drink, and swallow (including medications and drugs).

Acids are already contained in some foods, such as rhubarb and lemons. Other acids form only when a food is being metabolized as a result of the breakdown of proteins (uric and phosphoric acids), fats (fatty acids, acetylacetic acids), carbohydrates (pyruvic and succinic acids), and so forth.

An analysis of your regular diet determines the proportion of acidifying to alkalizing foods. If your intake of alkaline elements is higher than your intake of acids, there is no risk to the body of losing its acid–alkaline balance. To the contrary, it will be greatly supported in its efforts to maintain this balance, thanks to the excess alkaline elements.

When your acid intake is higher than that of your alkaline intake, however, your acid–alkaline equilibrium is dangerously compromised, and the body receives little of the assistance it needs to restore balance from the foods it consumes. It is then obliged to find a balance on its own using its own regulatory systems—in other words, by oxidizing, transporting, and eliminating excess acids.

The food analysis test is useful to verify whether the quantity of acidifying foods you're eating is higher or lower than that of alkaline foods. To do this, you need to establish a daily menu most representative of your usual diet.

To do a food analysis, keep a food diary, noting everything you consume in the course of a twenty-four-hour period. Be sure to include beverages and such incidentals as bread and between-meal snacks. Over the course of a few weeks you should notice patterns in your eating that could likely be described as two or three main menus.

In the sample menus provided below, the time of the meal is arbitrary; it serves only to distinguish between the various meals of the day. The variations possible during a particular meal are separated by the word "OR." There is no need to get lost in the details. For example, it is sufficient to note "cooked vegetables" or "raw vegetables," because (unless it is tomatoes) whether these vegetables are cabbage or carrots, they are alkaline foods, and that is what concerns us here. On the other hand, "beverage" or "dessert" is too imprecise, because a beverage or dessert is either acidifying or alkalizing depending on its composition. Likewise, there is no need to make a distinction between beef, pork, and chicken, but it is important to note whether the protein source for a meal is meat or cheese or eggs. Also, you don't need to measure quantities precisely; approximations are fine.

To indicate which foods belong to which group, in the example below acidifying foods are in *italic type*, alkalizing foods are in normal type, and acid foods are in **bold type**. Lists of these three different kinds of foods can be found on pages 52, 57, and 60, respectively.

EXAMPLES OF STANDARD MEALS

| 6:30 A.M. | EITHER | 1 large glass of water with **lemon** |
| | OR | *black coffee* |

7:00 A.M.	EITHER	*whole grain bread* (3 slices) + butter + *jelly* + 2 *coffees* + milk + 2 teaspoons *sugar* per cup
	OR	*cereal flakes* + milk + piece of **fresh fruit** + mint tea with no sugar
	OR	**plain yogurt** + **orange juice**

9:00 A.M.	EITHER	**apple**
	OR	*coffee* + *croissant*
	OR	half a *chocolate bar*
	OR	almonds + raisins
Beverage:	EITHER	1 quart of water in the morning
	OR	*2 or 3 coffees* + cream + *sugar*

Noon	EITHER	*meat dish* + *grain dish* +vegetable + *custard* + *coffee* + cream + *sugar*
	OR	*ham sandwich* + *glass of soda*
	OR	*cereal* + cooked vegetables + salad
	OR	*fish* + potatoes + raw vegetables + **fresh fruit**
Beverage		water OR *wine* OR *lemonade* OR *soda*
	OR	herb tea without sugar

4:00 P.M.	EITHER	*bread* + *chocolate* (pain au chocolat)
	OR	*pastry* + *coffee*
	OR	*cracker* + *tea* + *teaspoon sugar*
	OR	*lemonade*
	OR	**fresh fruit**
	OR	dried fruits + water

7:00 P.M.	EITHER	*two-egg omelet* + *brown bread* + green salad
	OR	homemade vegetable soup + *crackers* + *Swiss cheese*
	OR	*cold cuts* + *white bread* + *wine*
	AND/OR	*fruit tart* + *whipped cream* + *coffee* + cream + sugar
9:00 P.M.	EITHER	*peanuts* OR almonds OR *crackers*
	OR	*glass of milk*
	OR	**plain yogurt**

Once you've established your standard menu the kinds of foods that predominate in your diet will be clear. If you have difficulty metabolizing acids, you should determine whether acid and acidifying foods outweigh alkaline foods. Otherwise you simply need to see whether your intake of acidifying foods is higher than your intake of alkalizing and acid foods (these latter two have an alkalizing effect on people with no metabolic problems with acids). Detailed analyses of standard menus are provided in chapter 5.

TEST 4: LIFESTYLE ANALYSIS

In addition to diet, the manner in which you live your daily life has an influence on your acid–alkaline balance. A lifestyle analysis test is not sufficient on its own, however, to determine whether your internal environment is acidified. It should be used only as a complement to the other tests.

Because it is difficult to determine with any certainty at what point a behavior or activity stops being beneficial and becomes acidifying, the chart below describes extremes of behavior.

ACIDIFYING VS. ALKALIZING LIFESTYLES

Acidifying	Alkalizing (maintaining acid–alkaline balance)
sedentary lifestyle	active lifestyle
takes the elevator	walks up the stairs
travels mostly by car	travels on foot as much as possible
passive hobbies	active leisure-time pursuits
spends most of the time indoors	spends much time outdoors
stressed	calm, takes his or her time
restless, always short on time	relaxed and organized
sleep-deprived	gets plenty of sleep
restless sleep, insomnia	sleeps soundly
smokes	does not smoke
pessimistic	optimistic
loses temper easily, irritable	serene, patient
aggressive, envious, jealous	confident, tranquil

TEST 5: EXPERIMENTAL VERIFICATION

If acidification of the body prompts the appearance of many physical and mental problems, deacidifying the internal environment should logically bring about their disappearance. Of course, such change takes place gradually, beginning with the recent, more superficial problems and continuing with more serious, deep-rooted conditions that are caused by lesions.

Rapidly removing superficial acid from the body—the

procedure explained here—will enable you to verify whether the problems you are experiencing are due to acidification of the internal environment. If the easily reversed conditions—such as nervous irritation, chronic fatigue, skin inflammation, red blotches, heartburn and similar sensations, itching, and so forth—diminish significantly or totally disappear after five to ten days of deacidification, then you can safely assume they were caused by acids. On the other hand, if this alkalization treatment does not bring about a noticeable improvement in your well-being, the problems are in all likelihood caused by something other than acidification of the internal environment.

Rapid, superficial deacidification can be achieved through a massive intake of alkaline minerals in the very easily assimilated form of alkaline citrates. The specified daily dosage of these alkaline supplements should bring an acid pH of 5 or 6 back to the normal value of 7 to 7.5.

The complete procedure is explained in detail in chapter 6. Briefly, you begin the test by taking a half-teaspoonful of powdered alkaline citrate concentrate three times a day, or three tablets before each meal with water, then gradually increase the dosage until your urinary pH has returned to 7 or 7.5. Once you have determined this ideal dosage, you should maintain it for the five to ten days. Taking a larger amount of alkaline citrates, so the urinary pH rises above 7.5, would be useless, because the body cannot utilize the excess. It will simply flush the alkalines out in the urine without benefiting from them.

If your urinary pH is higher than 7 you should also perform this test, because, as explained earlier, a urinary pH with a reading higher than 7 does not necessarily mean that the internal environment of the body is not acid. The dosage of alkaline citrates should be set at two teaspoonfuls of powder three times a day or six tablets three times a day.

Rapid improvement of the problems from which you have been suffering means your body is ill because of a lack of alkaline elements, which is making your body's internal environment acid.

TEST 6: DETECTING INABILITY TO METABOLIZE ACIDS

This test is specifically indicated to determine if you have a metabolic inability to handle acids. It is based on the same principles as the previous test, but instead of taking alkaline supplements you temporarily increase your intake of acid foods—not *acidifying* foods, but acid foods such as fruits, vinegar, and whey. The acids from these foods are the most poorly metabolized by people suffering from this deficiency, so increasing intake of these acids will cause such people to experience temporary discomfort.

The purpose of this "challenge" test is not to make you sick, but simply to confirm or rule out the possibility that you have a deficiency in metabolizing acids. If you do, a more significant intake of acids should cause joint pains to intensify, red blotches on the skin to grow larger, fatigue to become more noticeable, and nervousness, burning urination, itching, and so forth to increase.

This test involves consuming generous helpings of fresh fruit, fruit juices, yogurts, whey products, and so forth for one or two days. This is long enough to bring about noticeable aggravation of symptoms. If you are extremely sensitive, the negative effects of acids may manifest as quickly as a half-hour to an hour after consumption. You will experience a general sense of feeling unwell and a sudden onset of fatigue, and your teeth may feel on edge in response to the aggressive acids.

Fortunately, it is not often necessary to perform this test. It is usually enough to recall what happened in the past under similar circumstances. For example, you may have seen negative effects after you ate a large quantity of fruit when it was in season, or a significant quantity of vinegar or yogurt. If you underwent a grape or lemon juice fast in the past, did it have a beneficial effect on your general health, restore your strength, and bring about the disappearance of illnesses? Or did it accentuate your symptoms and reduce your vitality?

In the first instance there is no case for a metabolic deficiency regarding acids, and it is clear that the primary causes for your state of acidification are acidifying foods and lifestyle choices. You can therefore eat acid foods, for they will have an alkalizing effect.

In the second instance, though, it would be clear that you have a metabolic weakness. You can assess the degree of the problem by the intensity of the aggravation of your symptoms. You should keep close watch not only over the quantity of acidifying foods in your diet, but also the amount of acid foods you consume.

Part Two

DIMINISHING ACIDIFICATION THROUGH DIET

3

Acidifying, Alkalizing, and Acid Foods

ᜑᜑᜑ

Diet is the principal source of the acid and alkaline substances that determine the acid–alkaline balance or imbalance of the body. It is therefore indispensable to have full knowledge of the properties of the foods you eat and to know precisely whether a given food has an alkalizing or acidifying effect on you personally.

In these next chapters, which are devoted to diet, the study of foods is presented in three stages.

This chapter begins with the three main groups into which food can be divided: acidifying foods, alkalizing foods, and acid foods. This is not the most common division—as a rule only the first two groups are distinguished—but, as explained previously, individuals with a metabolic inability to handle acids need to be able to distinguish *acidifying* from *acid* foods.

The acidifying or alkalizing nature of foods can vary enormously within one food category—for example, between different fruits and grains. Chapter 4 takes a more intensive look at these differences, tackling each kind of food and drink in turn and defining its strong, average, or weak acidifying qualities more precisely, so you can make a more judicious selection of foods when establishing your daily menus.

Chapter 5 examines menus for different meals, starting with a look at which menus for these meals—breakfast, snack, lunch, afternoon snack, and dinner—are now most common, and exploring their generally acidifying nature. This is followed by sample alkaline menus for good meals that will help restore the ideal acid–alkaline balance.

All the foods we eat can be divided into three basic groups: acidifying foods, alkalizing foods, and acid foods. The definitions of the first two groups are based on the effects these foods have on the body—either acidifying or alkalizing—whereas the criterion for the third group is based on a basic property of the food—specifically its acid flavor—and does not consider its effect on the body. What is the reason for this difference?

As much as possible the characteristics of foods should always be defined based on their effects on the body rather than their intrinsic qualities, as it is the effects that concern people who are concerned about their health. In fact, a food can display alkaline characteristics yet have an acidifying effect on the body. This is the case with white sugar, which is used to moderate the acid in the highly acidic tastes of certain fruits such as rhubarb or black currant. While this neutralization is very real on the level of taste, it vanishes when it comes to the body. When metabolized, white sugar produces numerous acids and is therefore strongly acidifying. In matters of therapeutic treatment it is very important to recognize the decisive nature of this effect.

A great mistake made by some dietitians is to consider only chemical analyses of foods and to assume that the body greatly benefits from the nutritive qualities revealed by these analyses.

The great French nutritionist and naturopath P. V. Marchesseau once said that "food has no intrinsic value. The only value it possesses comes from the digestive tract that receives it." How should we define the quality of a food such as grass, for example, when it is good or bad depending on whether it enters the digestive tract of a cow or a human being? The same holds true for foods appropriate for people: raw vegetables are good for someone in good health, but not for a patient with enteritis or colitis. For the latter, the coarse nature of the vegetable fiber causes even greater irritation to an already inflamed digestive tract. Dairy products are beneficial for most people, but not for those who are lactose intolerant, and so forth.

Knowing the effects a food has on the body is of fundamental importance. The foods in the first two groups, acidifying and alkalizing, have been classified according to their observed effects on human beings.

The effect of foods in the third group, that of acid foods, cannot be clearly defined in a definitive manner, unlike the first two groups. It varies according to the individual body's ability to metabolize acids. These foods, primarily fruits, whey, and vinegar, have an alkalizing effect on those whose bodies properly metabolize weak acids, but are acidifying for those whose bodies metabolize acids poorly if at all. As these foods cannot be classified according to their effects, they are defined by their intrinsic characteristic of acid taste.

Generally speaking, the foods from this group are associated with foods that have alkalizing qualities, because that is their effect on the majority of people who eat them. But it would be a serious error to adopt that as the sole classification, because, on the one hand, it does not entirely correspond to the reality, and on the other, most people who are concerned about their acid–alkaline balance have a metabolic weakness toward acids. For them, knowledge of this third group is crucial.

Understanding these three groups permits you to select without risk of error the foods that are necessary to add to your diet to restore the ideal acid–alkaline balance. You should choose foods according to these two rules of thumb:

- If your body metabolizes acids properly, **the quantity of alkalizing and acid foods should be higher than the quantity of acidifying foods.**

- If you have a metabolic inability to handle acids, **the quantity of alkalizing foods should be higher than the quantity of acidifying and acid foods.**

Two points need to be emphasized. First, the more a person is afflicted by acidification or a metabolic inability to handle acids, the higher should be the proportion of alkalizing foods in the diet in proportion to the others. In fact, while a person with a healthy acid–alkaline balance can eat acidifying and alkaline foods in equal amounts, people with an imbalance should make alkalizing foods 60 to 80 percent of their diet.

Reducing acidifying foods drastically or eliminating them completely would not be wise, because foods rich in proteins (eggs, dairy products, meat, fish) are among the acidifying group. An adequate intake of proteins is a prerequisite for alkaline minerals to establish themselves properly in the tissues. Tissues require proteins to produce a good framework to contain the minerals. Otherwise, a portion of the alkaline minerals ingested will leave the body and will therefore be unavailable when the body needs them to neutralize acids.

Second, the more you suffer from problems caused by acidification or a metabolic inability to handle acids, the greater the necessity to consume a more significant amount of alkaline foods *at every meal.* If you include those foods in every meal of the day, neutralization of food acids or acids produced in the digestive process is handled directly by the alkaline elements contributed by the food just eaten.

This intake represents a valuable aid to the body, for without it food acids leave the intestinal tract and enter the internal environment, forcing the body to draw from its tissue reserves the alkaline elements it requires to neutralize them. This results in a depletion of the body's mineral content and prompts the appearance of health conditions caused by acidification.

People who can metabolize acids properly are less subject to the necessity of eating more alkaline foods than acid foods. They have good reserves of alkaline elements that can be drawn on when needed to neutralize the acids from a meal that consists exclusively or almost exclusively of acidifying foods.

ACIDIFYING FOODS

Acidifying foods are primarily those that are rich in proteins, carbohydrates, and/or fats.

ACIDIFYING FOODS

- Meat, poultry, cold cuts, meat extracts, fish, seafood (mussels, shrimp)
- Eggs

- Cheeses (strong cheeses are more acidic than mild cheeses)
- Animal fats such as lard and suet
- Vegetable oils, especially peanut oil and oils that are refined or hardened (margarine)
- Whole grains and refined grains: wheat, oats, especially millet
- Bread, pasta, cereal flakes, and foods with a grain base
- Leguminous plants such as peanuts, soybeans, white beans, broad beans
- White sugar
- Sweets: syrups, pastry, chocolate, candy, jelly, fruit preserves
- Oleaginous fruits: walnuts, hazelnuts, pumpkin seeds
- Commercially manufactured sweet drinks, primarily sodas
- Coffee, tea, cocoa, wine
- Condiments such as mayonnaise, mustard, and ketchup

Foods rich in proteins (meat, dairy products, and leguminous plants) are acidifying because their digestion produces amino acids; and because proteins, once they have been utilized by the body's cells, engender products of acidic degradation, such as uric acid, which primarily comes from the proteins that serve in the construction of the cell core and are found in foods consisting of cells, such as animal meats. Unlike meat and fish, dairy products do not carry uric acid because milk and cheese are not composed of animal tissues. Furthermore, the essential amino acids that make up animal meats always contain phosphorus and sulfur, two acid minerals.

Although they are not composed of animal tissue, the

leguminous plants (soybeans, chickpeas) bring a large quantity of uric acid into the body because they are rich in purines. Intrinsically alkaline, these purines are transformed into uric acid so they may be eliminated from the body. The presence of large amounts of purines in coffee, tea, and cocoa also explains why these beverages, as well as chocolate, are acidifying.

The acidifying nature of foods rich in fats (animal fat used in cooking, the fat contained in meat, deep-frying oil) is twofold. First, fat is utilized by the body in the form of *fatty acids,* and secondly, *saturated* fatty acids—which animal-based foods contain in great quantity—are difficult to metabolize. When their digestion is incomplete they create toxic acid substances such as acetones, acetylacetic acid, beta-hydroxybutyric acid, and others. These waste products and metabolic residues appear only if fat breakdown in the body is faulty; normal digestion of fats yields fatty acids. As fat consumption is rather high in today's standard diet, acidification from fats is all too common.

The acidifying properties of carbohydrates are due to the same types of processes that are involved with fat and its acidic nature. In the form of starch, carbohydrates are actually aggregates of thousands of glucose molecules—up to 250,000 of them—whereas it takes only several hundred amino acids to produce a protein. For the body to use carbohydrates they must be broken down into increasingly smaller fragments until they are reduced to their basic constituent element: the glucose molecule.

The greatest culprit in the production of acids is the poor conversion of long chains of glucose. Just like fat and proteins, carbohydrates go through various stages of transformation during which their characteristic properties change what was originally alkaline into an acid. If these conversions are interrupted while in progress the body becomes acidified, because the intermediary acid substances are not converted back into alkaline substances, as would be the normal end result of this process. This breakdown of the process is all too common, since the overconsumption of carbohydrates (bread, cereals, pastas, crackers) is quite significant and often goes well beyond the body's capacity to digest them properly. The problem is the same whether the process involves whole grains or refined grains.

While cereal grains are acidifying, germinated grains are not. In fact, because of the radical transformation of their composition due to the germination process, these foods are considered to be alkalizing and are classified with green vegetables, since young grain sprouts are more or less green when eaten. This is also the case for the sprouts of leguminous plants such as soybeans, lentils, and chickpeas. (Bread made with sprouted grains, however, is not alkalizing.)

White sugar, a carbohydrate that consists of only two molecules (glucose and fructose), is acidifying for a different reason. Its acidifying nature, and that of the foods containing it (jellies, candies, chocolate, cookies), comes from the fact that it is refined and stripped of all trace elements, vitamins, and enzymes; it is thus generally poorly converted by the body. The body cannot indefinitely continue releasing large quantities of vitamins and trace elements to produce the conversion of sugar into energy. The average annual consumption of white sugar today is more than ninety pounds per person, which is more than the body can handle. The transformation of sugar in the body inevitably stalls at one of the intermediary acidic stages.

Refined white sugar and all the products that contain it are strongly acidifying, but the naturally occurring sugars of fruits and vegetables (like carrots and beets) are not. This is because the tissues of fruits and vegetables contain all the necessary trace elements, vitamins, and enzymes necessary to complete their transformation in the body. For the same reasons, whole sugar, meaning the concentrate obtained from the evaporation of sugar-cane sap, is not acidifying either. Brown sugars, on the other hand, have undergone several refining processes that have depleted their vitamin and trace element content. Consequently, they too are acidifying, and the closer they are to white sugar (the most acidic form of sugar), the more acidifying their effect is on the body. The fructose or fruit sugar available for sale commercially is also depleted of all its naturally occurring vitamin content, making it an acidifying agent as well.

Oleaginous fruits (except for almonds and Brazil nuts) are all acidifying, including walnuts, hazelnuts, cashews, pecans, coconut, or even the seeds used in health food mixes—sunflower seeds, pumpkin seeds, sesame seeds, and so forth. Their acidifying character is due to their high fat content as well as their high content of protein, phosphorus, and sulfur. However, a couple of sunflower seeds does not acidify the body to the same extent as six to twelve ounces of meat, although both foods are included in the list of acidifying foods.

Based on their characteristics, the foods in the acidifying group have an acidifying effect on everyone who eats them, unlike acid foods, which may have an acidifying or alkalizing effect depending on the individual's physical capabilities. The manner in which the body utilizes acidifying foods inevitably leads to the production of acids, so it is advisable to pay strict attention to the amount of acidifying foods you include in your daily diet if you want to avoid acidification of your internal environment. This does not mean an extreme reduction or complete elimination of these items from the diet; it is simply a matter of keeping the quantity of acidifying foods lower than that of alkalizing foods. This should be a general guideline for what you eat every day, or even better, for what you eat at every meal.

ALKALIZING FOODS

Alkalizing foods consist primarily of green and colored vegetables (with the exception of tomatoes) and potatoes.

These foods are alkalizing because they are rich in alkaline elements and contain little if any acid substances, and because they do not produce acids when they are utilized by the body. Even when significant amounts of this type of food are consumed, no acid is produced, regardless of the metabolic capacities of the person who eats them. Just as acidifying foods are acidifying for everyone, alkalizing foods are alkalizing for everyone. These are the foods that people suffering from an acid–alkaline imbalance need to eat above all.

Green and colored vegetables are the primary source of alkaline substances for the body. They should be included in every main meal, whether as salad, raw or cooked vegetables, juice, or soup, by anyone trying to restore or maintain acid–alkaline balance. The sole exception is the tomato, which is very acidifying whether eaten raw or cooked. (Botanically speaking, however, the tomato is not a vegetable but a fruit.)

ALKALIZING FOODS

- Potatoes
- Green vegetables, raw or cooked: salad greens, green beans, cabbage, and so on

- Colored vegetables: carrots, beets (except for tomatoes)
- Corn (kernels or cooked as polenta)
- Milk (liquid and powdered form), large-curd cottage cheese, cream, butter
- Bananas
- Almonds, Brazil nuts
- Chestnuts
- Dried fruits: dates, raisins (except for those that are acidic to the taste—apricots, apples, pineapple)
- Alkaline mineral waters
- Almond milk
- Black olives preserved in oil
- Avocado
- Cold-pressed oils
- Natural sugar

Potatoes are well known for their anti-acidifying qualities; their juice is often recommended as a remedy for stomach acidity and ulcers. The potato's wealth of alkaline elements makes it the best choice of foods to counter the acidification of the body. A starchy food, it is nourishing and a beneficial alternative to cereal grains, which are acidifying. A deacidifying diet must include potatoes more often than foods from cereal grains.

Another nourishing and valuable food for fighting excess acidity is the chestnut. Like the potato, it is starchy, a food that supplies fuel for energy, and it is not acidifying like cereal grains. Chestnuts can be roasted in the oven or boiled in water and eaten as a vegetable. The best-known recipe containing them is probably red cabbage with chestnuts. Like potatoes, chestnuts go well with cheese. But watch out for chestnut purees, which are often sweetened with sugar.

Of all the fruits, the banana is the only one that is truly alkalizing, because its own acid content is so weak that it never causes acidification, even when consumed in large quantities or as a regular part of the diet. Other fruits, in contrast, even those that are only faintly acid, such as melons, do contain acids, which means that the more one eats of them, the greater the acidifying effect they have.

Generally speaking, dried fruits (dates, raisins) are alkalizing because a portion of their acid content is oxidized in the drying process. They are less alkalizing if they are set out to dry before reaching full maturity, as is often the case with apples and apricots. The alkaline nature of dried fruits is also slightly reduced when they are treated with sulfur as a preservative.

Almonds and Brazil nuts are the only alkalizing oleaginous fruits. They can be eaten just as they are, or chopped or sliced and mixed with salads, vegetables, and desserts. Some dietetic and health food stores sell a sugarless almond paste, which can be mixed with water to make almond milk, a very pleasant and alkalizing beverage.

Black olives preserved in olive oil are alkalizing, unlike those, either black or green, that are preserved in a vinegar-based brine.

Raw or whole sugar is not alkalizing, properly speaking, meaning that it does not alkalize the internal environment if eaten in large quantities, but when eaten in moderation it does not acidify either, as is the case with other sugars. The same is true of corn, milk, large-curd cottage cheese, cream, butter, and so on, which, eaten in moderation, do not acidify the body.

Water usually has a pH of 7. When it is highly chlorinated, it becomes acid. Carbonated mineral water is also acid, because the gas that gives it its carbonation is carbonic acid. The principal alkaline mineral waters—those with a pH above 7—are Limpia Water (Italy), Contrexéville and Évian (France), and Henniez bleue (Switzerland). To determine whether a mineral water is alkaline, read the label on the bottle, as the pH is indicated there.

ACID FOODS

This group consists of foods whose alkalizing or acidifying effect depends on the metabolic capacities of the person who eats them. Their classification is therefore not based upon their physical effect (because that cannot be defined in advance) but on their basic nature, which is acid.

These foods contain a good deal of acid, hence their taste. The acids in them are weak, however, which means for people capable of metabolizing them properly by easily oxidizing them, they are transformed into alkaline elements and therefore contribute to the alkalization of the body. But for people whose metabolisms cannot handle acids properly, the large quantity of acids contained in these foods is not oxidized, and they thus will have an acidifying effect.

The primary acid foods are fruits, whey, and vinegar.

ACID FOODS

- Whey, yogurt, curds, kefir, small-curd cottage cheese
- Unripe fruits (the less ripe a fruit, the higher its acid content)
- Acid fruits: berries (red and black currants, raspberries, strawberries); citrus fruits (lemons, grapefruit, tanger-

ines, oranges); certain varieties of apples (Winesap), cherries (Morello), plums, apricots

- Sweet fruits (especially when eaten in excess), melon, watermelon
- Acid vegetables: tomato, rhubarb, sorrel, watercress
- Sauerkraut, vegetables that have been lactofermented (cultured with *Lactobacillus*)
- Fruit juices, lemon juice (in salad dressing)
- Honey
- Vinegar

The faintly acid taste of apples and pears, or the strongly acidic flavor of lemons and red currants, is indicative of how high or low their acid content is. For these foods the sense of taste can be used to determine the degree of acidity. The acid content is higher in unripe fruit: the less ripe it is, the more acid. Fruits that are perfectly ripe have the least acidity. Apricots, for example, are extremely acid before maturity, even if their color is already orange, but are alkaline when they become ripe and mellow. Even within a single species of fruit, for example apples or cherries, the degree of acidity of the fruit varies according to the variety; Winesap apples are more acidic than golden apples, Morello cherries are more acidic than Bing cherries, and so forth.

Drinking fruit juice as an alternative to eating the flesh of the fruit does not reduce the acid; on the contrary. Alkaline minerals are primarily located in the pulp and remain there when the fruits are pressed for juice. Since they are not present in the juice, they cannot neutralize its acidity. (This is, of course, not the case for juices that contain pulverized pulp.)

The consumption of fruits in the form of juice can also distort your impression of how much fruit you are eating. You probably do not eat more than two oranges at one sitting, but you can easily drink two or three glasses of orange juice at a time, the equivalent of six to eight oranges.

Cooking fruits also does not diminish their acidity. In the majority of cases, cooking simply increases the acidity because the heat destroys some of the vitamins and enzymes. Furthermore, most cooked fruit dishes have white sugar added, and we have already discussed the highly acidic properties of that food.

The case of whey is unique. This food, which consists of the liquid part of milk that has been curdled through fermentation, is a transparent, clear yellow liquid. It is found in fresh white cheeses like cottage or farmer cheese, yogurt (whey is the liquid that collects in the impression made by a spoon in yogurt), kefir, and so on. When fresh, whey is alkaline, but after an hour or two it becomes acid. It primarily creates lactic acid, which, like the acids found in fruits, is relatively easy for the body to oxidize and convert into an alkaline substance, so long as the individual has no trouble metabolizing acids. When there is a metabolic inability to handle acids, however, the acids are not converted and therefore contribute to the acidification of the body's internal environment. People with this metabolic deficiency have to monitor their intake of whey, yogurt, and kefir just as they do that of fruits.

The acid fermentation used to make yogurt can also be used to preserve vegetables or juices. Sauerkraut, lactofermented vegetables and vegetable juices, and vinegar, for the same reasons that apply to the foods we have just discussed, are acidifying for those with metabolism difficulties with acids but are alkalizing for everyone else.

Honey is moderately acidic.

The acidifying or alkalizing nature of fruits, whey, and vinegar is the subject of constant debate. Of course, people whose metabolisms have no problem with acids are convinced of the alkalizing nature of these foods, while the rest remain equally convinced of their acidifying nature based on their personal experience. There is no reason for this controversy ever to have arisen. These foods can either be acidifying or alkalizing, and as such they form a distinct third group that has been defined as acid foods.

In cases of extreme acidification, there is no need to worry that the total removal of all fruits from the diet will result in an insufficient intake of vitamins, as some have claimed. Fruit is certainly an extraordinary source of vitamins, but vegetables contain many as well, quite a broad spectrum, in fact. Because vegetables are the foundation of the diet of those suffering from acidification, the amount they consume should cover their daily vitamin requirements.

In fact, the elimination of acid foods will not cause major problems, because none of them are absolutely indispensable, unlike some foods with acidifying properties. Fresh fruits can be replaced with dried fruits, dairy products rich in whey by those containing none, and lactofermented vegetables by fresh vegetables. In practice, it is often necessary for a person suffering from this kind of metabolism deficiency to completely eliminate acid foods from the diet for several weeks to a month. This restriction has never created problems (other than the person's yearning to eat a food from this group that she or he enjoys). But the benefits of the deacidification more than compensate for the temporary sacrifice.

EIGHT RULES FOR AN ACID–ALKALINE BALANCED DIET

There are four elementary principles for selecting foods to ensure the proper quantities of acidifying, alkalizing, and acid foods in the diet. These are accompanied by four additional rules to be followed by people who are unable to metabolize acids properly.

- Rule one: A meal should never consist solely of acidifying foods but should always contain alkaline foods.

A meal of meat with pasta, or fish and rice, with cake and coffee for dessert is not a recommended menu because it consists entirely of acidifying foods; the same applies to a meatless meal of pasta with tomato sauce followed by a dessert sweetened with white sugar. By adding vegetables to this meal in the form of salads or raw or cooked vegetables, the alkaline intake at least partially compensates for the acids. Vegetables are typically included with meals, but often in such small quantities that their effect is negligible. This takes us to rule number two.

- Rule two: The amount of alkalizing foods should be greater proportionately than the amount of acidifying foods at any one meal.

The proportion of foods that produce alkaline elements

should always be greater than that of foods that produce acids. Eating in this manner ensures that the acids are neutralized at the intestinal or tissue level without any need for the body to draw from its reserves.

- Rule three: The proportion of alkalizing foods should be even greater proportionately when there is pronounced acidification of the internal environment or when the individual is unable to metabolize acids properly.

The more the body is weakened or exhausted, the less alkaline reserve it has for its buffer system, and the less capable it is of oxidizing acids. Putting less acid into the body makes it easier for the body to maintain its acid–alkaline balance.

- Rule four: A diet consisting solely of alkaline vegetables and plant-based food is possible, but only for a limited period (one to two weeks).

An exclusively alkaline diet, consisting solely of vegetables, potatoes, bananas, almonds, and so forth, cannot be continued indefinitely because it is seriously inadequate in protein. Such diets are useful when acidification is very significant and the disorders it has caused are acute, intense, and painful. The abrupt, complete elimination of all acids allows the body to recover more rapidly and return to a normal acid–alkaline balance. An exclusively alkaline diet should remain a short-term therapeutic action so as not to compromise health.

There are four additional rules that people suffering from an inability to metabolize acids properly should heed.

- Rule five: A meal should never consist solely of acid foods but should always include alkaline foods.

This rule is almost identical to rule one, but it involves acid rather than acidifying foods. Eating fruits and yogurt exclusively or drinking only whey-based beverages is strongly discouraged, as the acid intake from such a diet is not compensated by any alkaline food, which forces the body to draw these substances from its own tissues. The risk of health problems caused by mineral depletion is therefore quite significant. These manifest as a sudden drop in vitality, the feeling that one's teeth are on edge, a chilly sensation, itching, joint pains, and others that have been discussed previously.

Alkaline foods that are good accompaniments to fresh fruits are fresh (unripened) cheeses, soft white cheese (large-curd cottage cheese, low-fat cream cheese, ricotta, quark, mozzarella, farmer cheese, fresh goat cheese, yogurt cheese), cream, almonds, bananas, salad greens, or a blend of raw fruits and vegetables.

- Rule six: The quantities of acid and acidifying foods a person eats should be tailored to meet their personal metabolic capabilities.

The inability to metabolize acids properly is rarely absolute; it varies according to individual physiology as well as circumstances (such as stress, fatigue, work, and vacations). Each person has a certain rate at which he or she can metabolize acids properly, a rate that cannot be surpassed without overtaxing the body's capacity.

As long as the quantity of acids ingested or created by the digestion of food is below these rates, the body manages to neutralize them through oxidation before any of the health problems created by acidification manifest. Accordingly, for certain extremely sensitive individuals, half a golden apple—no more—suits them just fine, but even a quarter of a Winesap apple is more than they can handle. For any given person, a certain quantity of a food can be acidifying, yet alkalizing or neutral in a lesser amount.

So if you have difficulty metabolizing acids, you can safely eat acid foods as long as you tailor the amount you consume to your physical capacities. Your tolerance threshold can also change over time. You can discover and keep track of your own threshold through experimentation and observation.

- Rule seven: Acid foods should not be eaten too rapidly in succession.

An individual with an inability to metabolize acids properly, but with a normal acid–alkaline balance, can generally handle a sudden increase in acid intake (from eating a large quantity of fruit, for example) by drawing from the body's reserves, provided that this kind of event is the exception and not the rule. In fact, if the withdrawal of alkaline substances from the body's reserves is a unique event, the acid–alkaline balance is not endangered, and no acidification problem will occur.

But some time will have to go by before the body's reserves are replenished. If eating another piece of fruit puts additional acids into the body too soon, it has to draw from its already diminished reserves, which may not contain enough alkaline substances to neutralize the acid from the fruit, and acid–alkaline balance is compromised. Health problems due to acidification will appear not because the body was not intrinsically capable of neutralizing this fruit's acid—it had successfully done so before—but because the fruit had been eaten too soon after the first fruit had been consumed.

By spacing out the ingestion of these hard-to-metabolize foods, you can increase your personal level of tolerance for them. This is useful to know, as it allows you to expand the selection of foods you can safely eat.

- Rule eight: Acid foods must be eaten when the body is ready to receive them.

There is an Arabic proverb that says: "Oranges are like gold in the morning, silver at noon, and lead in the evening." For people with an inability to metabolize acids properly, the opposite is true. Oranges and fruits in general are harmful in the morning and much more beneficial at noon or in the evening. The reason for this is that by noon the body's "organic motor" has had the time to warm up and is turning over naturally. In fact, some people take a long time *physically* to wake up in the morning. The heart beats more slowly, blood pressure is low, and cellular exchanges—including oxidation—take place in slow motion. The body reaches cruising speed only after several hours of activity and a meal or two. If such a person eats fruits or drinks a glass of orange juice in the morning, not only will he or she have difficulty metabolizing the acids but, because the body is still working below its real capacity, it will have even greater trouble oxidizing acids than it normally would.

Along the same lines of reasoning, acids foods are metabolized better in the summer, when the weather is hot and sunny, as well as when one is rested (as opposed to feeling tired).

4

Classifying the Acidification Potential of Foods

ॐ

In the previous chapter we divided food into three basic categories. Even within a single category, however, not all foods are uniformly alkalizing, acidifying, or acid. For example, both rice and millet are acidifying foods, but millet is much more acidifying than rice. To fine-tune an optimal diet, we need to refine these classifications.

The classification used here presents foods in a three-column chart. Alkaline foods are divided into strongly alkalizing, weakly alkalizing, and acidifying. Acid foods are categorized as alkalizing, weakly acidifying, and strongly acidifying. This division helps people suffering from acidification avoid inadvertently choosing only weakly alkalizing foods when they could just as easily eat strongly alkalizing foods, which are of much greater benefit in correcting the imbalance of their internal environment.

This is not a precise hierarchical organization, where each food occupies a set place with regard to the others; we currently lack the objective criteria necessary for establishing such an exact hierarchy. Analysis of a food's chemical composition is not germane because it does not take into account what happens once the food has been ingested. As we have seen, digestion and the body's utilization of foods alter their properties. These classifications are therefore based on observation of the effects these foods have on the body.

Based on your own experience, however, you may feel one food or another is better placed in a category different than the one assigned to it here. This is not surprising, since each person's body has its own strengths and weakness in handling certain foods. It can in fact be the case that a food has a very acidifying effect on one person, whereas for most people its acidifying effect is weak. You are well advised to trust your own experience rather than to base all your food choices on theory.

Nonetheless, the classification on these charts is valid for the majority of people. For the rest, it can serve as a useful guide for taking the first steps while they are in the process of determining how to modify their diet according to their individual needs and the intrinsic capabilities of their own bodies.

FRESH FRUITS

The classification of fresh fruits is valid only for those who are unable to metabolize acids properly. For everyone else, all fruits have an alkalizing effect.

Because a fruit's acidifying properties depend on how ripe it is—the more ripe, the less acid—the classification assumes the fruits listed are in their ripest state. But just what is a ripe fruit, exactly?

Most people today do not have gardens or orchards, so they depend on grocery stores for their produce. But for economic reasons, most fruit sold in stores is harvested long before it reaches maturity, because fruit is less fragile (and therefore easier to ship) when still hard and green. The spoilage rate is therefore greatly reduced, and the fruit can survive the elaborate handling that takes place at the level of the producer, the wholesaler, the retail seller, and finally the consumer. Picking fruit when it is unripe also permits better management of inventory, as the flow of merchandise can easily be adapted to the needs of the market.

The harmful result of this premature harvesting is that fruit never reaches the full ripeness that makes it soft, aromatic, sweet, and juicy. If you have ever had the opportunity to taste a fruit that has ripened on the tree in the open air, bathed in the rays of the sun, you know how much more delicious it is than what you usually eat.

Aside from the question of taste, the natural ripening of fruits brings about very significant reduction in their acid content, much more than takes place in fruits harvested before they are ripe. One of my patients, who could not metabolize acids properly, loved oranges but could not eat them without experiencing discomfort. To his great surprise, when he took a trip to an orange-producing region just at the time the fruit was ripe, he found he could eat a pound or more of oranges daily without the least bit of distress. Having attained their full maturation under the sun rather than sitting in a warehouse since they were green, these oranges now contained only a very small amount of acids, which were quite easy for him to metabolize.

Every fruit is a complete entity in and of itself and should whenever possible be eaten in its entirety, skin and seeds and all. Of course, apricot kernels and cherry stones are too large to be swallowed easily and too hard to be digested. But apple, orange, and grape seeds, among others, contain elements that are of great benefit to the body and are useful to its metabolism of the fruit. Furthermore, the skin of fruits contains numerous minerals and enzymes that facilitate neutralization of the acid contained in the fruit pulp. It is thus a mistake to peel apples and pears and to get rid of the skins of figs, grapes, prunes, and so forth. Only orange and citrus fruit peel, melon rind, and pomegranate skin should be thrown away, even if they have not been treated with pesticides and other chemicals.

Fresh fruits can be eaten as they are or shredded or chopped in a fresh fruit salad. Fresh fruits are naturally sweet, so adding sugar should be avoided, because sugar is an acidifying agent. It is also best not to eat fruits along with cereal grains—for example, in granola or muesli—because the combination of fresh fruit and cereal flakes is hard to digest and encourages fermentation, which is a great producer of acid toxins.

Cooking fruit does not reduce its acidity. When cooking compotes and pies, it is important to use ripe apples and not green apples that have fallen prematurely.

Shredding or slicing fruit makes it more alkaline, because the contact of the pulp with air allows some of its acid content to oxidize.

The only alkalizing fruit, the banana, is not easily digested by everyone. This is usually because it has been picked before it has become truly ripe. A ripe banana has very sweet, soft flesh. Its sugar content can be increased by mashing it into a puree with a fork or spoon and allowing it to sit out in the air for ten to twelve minutes before eating it.

Another way to neutralize the aggressive nature of fruit-based acids is to eat them with soft white cheese, fresh cheese,

FRESH FRUITS

Alkalizing	Slightly acidifying	Very acidifying
	FRUITS	
	Golden Delicious apples	cider, Winesap apples
	pears: Bartlett, Comice, Bosc, Seckel	other pears
	grapes	
	plums	nectarines, greengage plums
	very ripe apricots	other apricots
	Bing cherries	Morello cherries
	peaches	
	figs	
	yellow plums (mirabelles)	
	melons	
	watermelon	
	BERRIES	
	strawberries, big and sweet	strawberries, small and tart
	gooseberries	red currants in bunches
	blueberries	raspberries
		black currants
		sea buckthorn
		sloe (blackthorn berries)
		mulberries
	CITRUS FRUITS	
	Clementines	mandarins
		oranges
		lemons
		citron
		grapefruit
	EXOTIC FRUITS	
bananas	mangos	pineapples
	pomegranates	kiwis
	persimmons	

or cream. This is common in many cuisines, as it is to eat smaller fruits such as strawberries and raspberries with crème fraîche or sour cream.

DRIED FRUITS

Dried fruits have lost the greater portion of their water content, and thus their juice, after having been set out to dry under the sun or in an oven. Dates are an exception; they are naturally low in water, and the way they appear in the stores ready for consumption is exactly how they look when ripening on the tree.

DRIED FRUITS

Alkalizing	Slightly acidifying	Very acidifying
raisins	prunes	tart apricots, sulfur-treated
sweet apricots,	pears	
dried naturally	apples	
bananas	peaches	
dates	figs	
	mangos	
	pineapple	

Because dried fruits are naturally quite sweet, they usually do not have sugar added to them before they are sold, with the exception of some dates that are packed in a sweet syrup.

Of course, the riper and sweeter a fruit is before it is dried, the higher its alkaline content after this process. The acidity of the fresh fruit is reduced in any event by the drying process thanks to oxidation.

Dried fruits play a very small role in the average diet of

most people, and many people never eat them. Because they are alkalizing, however, their consumption ought to be encouraged. They allow individuals with a high sensitivity to the acids of fresh fruits to eat fruit in a form suitable for their particular needs.

Dried fruit is extremely concentrated, and some people have trouble digesting it. Soaking the fruit in water for twelve to twenty-four hours before eating it makes it more easily digestible. It can be eaten with or without its soaking liquid.

Soaked dried fruit can also be made into delicious desserts by blending the fruit and its soaking liquid with a fromage blanc or cream cheese.

OLEAGINOUS FRUITS

As the name suggests, oleaginous fruits are rich in oil. Half their weight, in fact, consists of oil. Many people consider them to be incidental rather than staple foods and only eat them occasionally when they are part of a cake or cookie.

Of all the oleaginous fruits, only two are truly alkaline: almonds and Brazil nuts. But the alkalizing benefits of almonds are so strong that people suffering from acidification should eat them on a regular basis. Black olives are equally alkalizing, in contrast to green olives, but only if they have been preserved in oil and not in a brine or vinegar preparation.

Oleaginous fruits can be eaten just as they are, either one variety at a time or in combination, or along with dried fruits. Because of their high concentrations of basic nutrients it is better not to mix too many different kinds together, as this can make them difficult to digest. Crushed, slivered, or grated oleaginous fruits can be added to fruit salads, green salads, and raw-vegetable platters, or can be spread on bread like butter. Many different kinds of nut butters and pastes are readily available in supermarkets, groceries, and gourmet and health food stores. Peanut butter sandwiches, of course, are a lunchbox staple. Non-sweetened almond paste can also be used to make almond milk. Tahini, or sesame paste, is an ingredient in many popular Middle Eastern dishes, such as hummus and baba ganoush.

OLEAGINOUS FRUITS

Alkalizing	Slightly acidifying	Very acidifying
almonds	cashews	walnuts
Brazil nuts	sesame seeds	hazelnuts
black olives in oil	pine nuts	peanuts
	coconut	pecans
	green olives	pistachios
		pumpkin seeds
		sunflower seeds
		olives in brine or vinegar

VEGETABLES

Except for tomatoes and eggplants, which are quite acidifying, all vegetables are alkalizing and should make up a significant portion of your diet if you are suffering from problems caused by acidification. Some vegetables are very alkalizing, however, and others are less so. The latter have been listed in a second column under the heading "Slightly alkaline"; these are chiefly white (endive, celery, cauliflower, etc.) and sulfurous vegetables.

Sulfurous, or cruciferous, vegetables (broccoli, Brussels sprouts, radishes, onions, peppers, etc.) can restore minerals to the depleted physical internal environment of a person suffering from acidification, but they also contain sulfur, which itself is acid. Among sensitive individuals the sulfur not only has a slightly acidifying effect but is also an irritant to the mucous membranes of the digestive system, as well as to the respiratory mucous membranes and the skin when the acid is eliminated, organs that are already weakened and sensitive in people suffering from acidification. But this is of concern only if you are overly sensitive to acids, and only when you consume too large a quantity of the vegetables in question.

White and sulfurous vegetables can therefore be eaten, but to guarantee a good supply of minerals it is best to eat primarily green and colored vegetables, potatoes, and certain fruiting vegetables (cucumber, sweet pepper, etc.)

Vegetables can be eaten raw, cooked, in soup, or in juice. When you eat them raw with a dressing, be sure the dressing is not so acidic that it destroys their beneficial alkalizing qualities. Too often, such dressings contain so much vinegar or lemon juice that they not only drown out the flavor of the vegetables, but are also strongly acidifying if you are unable to metabolize acids properly. In that case you need to measure your intake of vinegar or lemon juice in teaspoons, not tablespoons. (Experiments have shown that vinegar is less acidifying than lemon juice.)

Cooked vegetables contain smaller amounts of vitamins than raw vegetables, because cooking destroys some of their vitamin content. However, the mineral content—which is most important in terms of restoring a healthy acid–alkaline balance—is not altered when vegetables are braised, steamed, or roasted. Boiling draws minerals from the vegetables into the cooking water, which is generally thrown away after use, along with these valuable elements.

Vegetables can make up part or all of a single meal. Homemade vegetable soup is highly recommended, especially in winter, for not only does it replenish the body's mineral content (soup contains the vegetables' mineral-rich cooking liquid), but its warmth counteracts one of the most common symptoms of acidification, the feeling of always being cold (due to the depletion of minerals).

Homemade vegetable juice has more benefit than canned, since it is fresh. Commercial vegetable juices vary in freshness, depending how they are preserved. If you have trouble metabolizing acids you should avoid juices that have been lactofermented, because they are slightly acidic.

If you make your own vegetable juice you can use a single vegetable or make a vegetable cocktail out of several different varieties. If possible, use organic produce so as to avoid ingesting chemicals. If the juice is too strong for your taste, you can dilute it with water without losing any of the alkalizing benefits. (Water has a neutral pH except when chlorinated, a process that makes it more acidic.)

VEGETABLES

Very alkaline	Slightly alkaline	Acidifying
potatoes		
GREEN VEGETABLES		
salad greens: chicory, escarole, lettuce, mâche, dandelion		
green cabbage		
celery stalks		
green beans		
fennel		

Very alkaline	Slightly alkaline	Acidifying
beet greens		
artichokes		
broccoli		
Brussels sprouts		

	COLORED VEGETABLES	
spinach		
carrots		
red beets		
red cabbage		
yellow beans		
sweet potatoes		

	FRUITING VEGETABLES	
edible gourds	avocado	tomato
zucchini		eggplant
squash		sour pickles
cucumber		
sweet pepper		

	WHITE VEGETABLES	
	endive	
	celeriac	
	salsify	
	Jerusalem artichoke	
	cauliflower	
	parsnip	
	Chinese artichoke	

	SULFUROUS VEGETABLES	
	radishes	
	turnips	
	peppers	
	onions	
	garlic	
	shallots	
	asparagus	

CEREAL GRAINS

There are countless ways to prepare cereal grains. They can be eaten whole (rice, spelt, etc.), ground (polenta, couscous, bulgur), crushed into cereal flakes, or ground into flour to thicken sauces and soups and to make bread, biscuits, and crackers, or very finely ground to be used in cakes and pastas.

With the exception of corn, all cereals and their by-products are acidifying. Their acidity increases in proportion to their refinement; white rice, for example, is much more acidifying than brown rice.

Of all the cereal grains, millet is the most acidifying. This is important to know, as it is often recommended for its excellent ability to replenish minerals in the case of hair loss, rheumatism, and so on because of its high silica content. However, silica is an acid mineral that is usually found in the form of silicic acid. Millet's ability to restore minerals to the body is undeniable, but people with problems digesting acid should avoid it, because its silica content is more than their bodies can deal with.

CEREAL GRAINS

Alkalizing	Slightly acidifying	Very acidifying
WHOLE GRAINS, GROUND GRAINS, GERMINATED GRAINS		
corn	wheat	millet
	brown rice	white rice
	rye	
	barley	
	spelt	
	buckwheat	
	quinoa	
	pilpil	couscous

Alkalizing	Slightly acidifying	Very acidifying
	whole semolina cream of rice	semolina
BREADS		
	whole-grain bread (without yeast) dark bread	yeast bread white bread
CRACKERS		
	whole grain	made from white flour
PASTA		
	whole grain	made from white flour
CEREAL FLAKES		
	whole-grain cereals, soaked for about 10 hours naturally baked flakes (e.g., corn flakes)	sugar frosted sweetened granola, muesli baked and sugared flakes
GRANOLA BARS		
	whole grain with little sugar	with lots of sugar and/or chocolate coated
COOKIES AND CAKES		
	whole grain with little sugar cake made from whole wheat	made with white flour, white sugar, chocolate cakes, pies white cake flour

White bread is more acidifying than whole-grain or dark breads because, stripped of vitamins, trace elements, and enzymes to make it more easily digestible, it produces—like white sugar—numerous acids. Yeast breads have also been included with acidifying foods, because the yeast that makes dough rise also makes it acidic, as can easily be verified by tasting it. It is still excellent bread, but it is difficult to metabolize for many people, especially those who are acid sensitive.

Toasting or grilling bread facilitates its digestion, because cooking cereal grains is the equivalent of predigesting them. Bread crust is more easily digested than the center portion, as the crust is more thoroughly cooked. Toasting bread slightly reduces its acidifying quality. For this same reason, crackers, which are all crust, are also less acidifying than freshly baked bread. Stale bread is less acidifying as well.

Cereal flakes that are crunchy (such as corn flakes) are less acidifying than those that are not (such as the oats used in muesli), because the former have been toasted.

The acidifying quality of pastas is typically made worse by the customary tomato sauce, tomatoes being the most acidifying vegetable. Pasta—preferably made from whole-grain flour—served plain, or with a white sauce or a little grated cheese, is a healthy alternative to pasta with tomato sauce.

Fruit pies and tarts combine several acidifying ingredients: flour, sugar, and fruit. The fruit used is often not ripe. It is better to eat such pastries only on occasion, and only when they have been made with ripe fruit. It is also a good idea to include grated or shredded almonds or cream to compensate for the acidity.

DAIRY PRODUCTS

Whole milk, whether raw or pasteurized, is alkalizing, but it becomes acidifying when it is sterilized, ultra-pasteurized, homogenized, and otherwise processed, because it then becomes increasingly difficult to metabolize. Although milk is naturally alkalizing, most adults have lost the digestive capacity they had as children to make milk curdle. Milk may be safely drunk in the form of a fruit-based milkshake or smoothie, because the acidity of the fruits causes the milk to curdle in the stomach. When chocolate and/or sugar are added, milk becomes an acidifying beverage.

Cheeses with either a hard or soft crust are acidifying. Their acidity increases in proportion to their fat content, their age, and how strong they are.

Well drained and eaten in moderation, cottage cheese and other soft unripe cheeses are slightly alkalizing. On the other hand, the more whey they contain, and the older they are, the more acid they become. (Large-curd cottage cheese tends to be better drained and thus more alkalizing than small-curd cottage cheese.) Furthermore, not only will their acidity increase, but their originally lactic levogyre L+ acids will be transformed into lactic dextrogyres D− acids. These acids are much harder to metabolize by the body, which cannot oxidize them properly due to the lack of the specific enzyme necessary to transform them. The greatest part of these acids is neither assimilated nor utilized by the body, but is directly eliminated in the urine in the hours immediately following their consumption. This elimination does not come without cost, however, since in order to neutralize the acidity, alkaline elements must be expended. Foods containing these kinds of lactic acids thus have a tendency to deplete the body's mineral content.

L+ lactic acid, in contrast, is very much in harmony with the body's physiology. The body transforms lactose to this form of lactic acid, and it is also what the muscles produce when burning sugar. When present in excess, L+ lactic acid causes aches and pains. The body does possess the necessary enzymes to transform L+ acid, so this substance does not have an acidifying effect.

In making yogurt, the proportion of L+ lactic acids can change completely depending on the method of fermentation used. Elevated levels of L+ lactic acid are found in the new varieties of yogurt that contain live cultures. Of course, the substantial amounts of sugar added to flavored yogurts make them acid.

Fresh butter, eaten raw and in moderation, is alkalizing, but it loses this advantage when eaten in large quantities or after being subjected to heat in cooking.

Eggs are slightly acidifying. Eaten alone, the yolk is alkalizing, however.

DAIRY PRODUCTS

Alkalizing	Slightly acidifying	Very acidifying
MILK PRODUCTS		
raw whole milk banana smoothie	pasteurized milk fruit smoothie crème fraîche	ultrapasteurized milk chocolate milk
BUTTER		
fresh butter		butter used in cooking (heated)
SOFT UNRIPENED CHEESES		
fresh, well drained	slightly drained	

Alkalizing	Slightly acidifying	Very acidifying
	CULTURED MILK PRODUCTS	
acidophilous milk	fresh yogurt	aged yogurt
	levrogyres yogurt	dextrogyre yogurt
	(*bifidus* live culture)	sweetened yogurt with
	yogurt drinks	fruit
	without sugar	kefir
fresh whey	slightly aged whey	aged whey
fresh buttermilk		aged buttermilk
	SOFT CHEESE	
	Camembert, Brie;	Same cheeses
	fresh young cheeses	but very ripe, old, with
	with little fat content	higher fat content
	HARD CHEESE	
	Swiss, Provolone	stronger flavored;
		Parmesan
	EGGS	
egg yolk	whole eggs	

MEAT AND FISH

Meats can be divided into two basic groups: white and red. The latter contain a higher quantity of toxins, blood, and fat, from which their deeper color is derived. But they also have a much higher acidifying effect on the body, the worst culprit being delicatessen meats and cold cuts. Fish is not much less acidifying than meat. Crustaceans (shrimp, crayfish), however, are even more acidifying, as are the majority of shellfish. Oysters are the one exception. Their high mineral content—minerals of all sorts, not simply alkaline minerals—make them an excellent source of minerals for building up the body's stores.

MEAT AND FISH

Alkalizing	Slightly acidifying	Very acidifying
MEAT		
	"white" meat: poultry, rabbit, veal, young lamb	"red" meat: beef, mutton, pork, cold cuts
FISH		
	lean fish: whiting, sole, flounder, trout, perch	fatty fish: salmon, carp, herring, mackerel
SEAFOOD		
oysters		crustaceans: lobster, shrimp, crayfish; mussels

LEGUMINOUS PLANTS (BEANS)

Leguminous plants are highly concentrated foods. They contain little water and consist almost entirely of proteins, lipids (fats), and glucides (carbohydrates). Peanuts, for example, contain 35 percent protein, 48 percent fat, and 25 percent glucides, leaving a mere 2 percent for water and mineral salts.

Leguminous plants are extremely potent acidifiers due to their high concentration of acidifying nutrients, and because they are rich in purines. For the body to eliminate this toxin it has to transform it into uric acid. One ounce of soybeans contains as many purines as two ounces of pork. Tofu and soy milk are much less acidifying because the process used to manufacture them makes them easier to metabolize.

LEGUMINOUS PLANTS (BEANS)

Alkalizing	Slightly acidifying	Very acidifying
SOYBEANS		
soy milk soy milk yogurt soybean sprouts	tofu	soybeans
OTHER BEANS		
	dried peas lentils kidney beans white beans navy beans	chickpeas (garbanzo beans) red beans peanuts

MISCELLANEOUS FOODS

Alkalizing	Slightly acidifying	Very acidifying
SUGAR		
raw cane sugar (Succanat) pear concentrate	maple syrup honey	white and brown sugar
SALT		
sea salt table salt		
SPICES AND CONDIMENTS		
green herbs: parsley, basil, etc.		capers pickles pimentos mustard mayonnaise ketchup
	apple cider vinegar	other kinds of vinegar

Alkalizing	Slightly acidifying	Very acidifying
OILS		
virgin cold pressed: sunflower, olive, safflower, etc.	same oils but heat pressed	peanut, walnut, hazelnut oils used in cooking (heated)
FATS		
nonhydrogenated vegetable margarine		hydrogenated margarine (palm or coconut oil) lard
MUSHROOMS		
	button mushrooms	other mushrooms: truffles, morels, etc.

BEVERAGES

Water—which should be the basic drink of every human being—generally has a pH of 7, but this can vary quite a bit depending on its origins. Tap water is usually acidic because it is most often chlorinated, and chlorine is an acid. Bottled mineral waters typically have a pH of 7, but if carbonated gas is added, as is the case with many popular brands, it becomes acidic. Slight carbonation decreases water's normal pH of 7 to 6 or 5.5, and high carbonation decreases it even further, to 5.

The most alkaline mineral waters I have found (this is by no means an exhaustive list) are Contrexéville (France), with a pH of 7.1; Évian (France), with a pH of 7.2; Henniez bleue (Switzerland), with a pH of 7.5; and Limpia (Italy), with a pH of 7.5 (although it is officially 7.99 right at the springs). The label on the mineral water bottle will indicate the water's pH.

For more information on the mineral content of waters you can consult the Web site www.mineralwaters.org.

The water filters sold commercially to purify tap water filter out the calcium and consequently acidify the water. Nevertheless, acidification of the body's internal environment is much less dependent on consumption of water—even of slightly acid water—than it is on other factors.

Coffee, tea, and chocolate drinks are acidifying because of their purine content. Herb teas and plant-based infusions such as mint, verbena, or linden blossom are alkalizing, except for those containing rose hips, fruit peels, and birch leaves. Horsetail, which is rich in silicic acid, like millet, has an acidifying effect on people whose metabolisms cannot cope with acids.

Juice made from ripe sweet fruits like mangoes or peaches is alkalizing if drunk in small quantities (one small glass a day). Other juices—mainly grapefruit and orange—have an acidifying effect on individuals whose metabolisms are deficient in dealing with acids.

Vegetable juices are alkalizing as a rule, unless they are preserved by lactofermentation. Tomato juice is always acidifying, however.

As noted earlier, whey is alkalizing or not depending on its age.

Commercial sodas, commercial brands of lemonade, and similar beverages are very acidifying because of their high sugar content.

BEVERAGES

Alkalizing	Slightly acidifying	Very acidifying
pure water		
MINERAL WATERS		
flat with a pH of 7: Contrexéville, Évian, Henniez bleue, Limpia	slightly carbonated	heavily carbonated
TAP WATER		
depending on source and how treated	depending on source and how treated	depending on source and how treated
FILTERED WATER (CHARCOAL FILTER)		
	old filter, 6.5 pH new filter, 6 pH	
COFFEE, TEA, HERB TEA		
coffee substitute mint tea, verbena, linden, etc.	green tea birchbark, rose hips, fruit peels	coffee black tea hot chocolate cocoa horsetail
JUICE		
fresh vegetables fresh whey almond milk soy milk	lactofermented vegetables slightly aged whey	tomato aged whey commercial lemonade sodas
ALCOHOL		
	beer	wine liqueurs, cordials strong spirits

5

Acidifying Meals and Alkalizing Alternatives

~

Most people choose their foods out of habit. You probably have no idea why you eat one way in preference to any other. If your eating habits are healthy, this should cause no problem. As soon as health problems appear, however, analyzing the way you eat will enable you to adjust your diet to be more balanced.

Countless people who suffer from acidification and the disorders it causes are eating highly acidifying meals without even being aware of it. The objective of this chapter is therefore to analyze the most common menus for the various meals and snack times of the day—breakfast, lunch, dinner, the ten o'clock coffee break, and the afternoon tea or snack break—to show their acidifying properties, and then to suggest some alkalizing alternatives.

The foods that make up the various menus and their suggested replacements are presented in three-column charts like those we used in the previous chapter. The columns make the same distinctions between alkalizing, slightly acidifying, and highly acidifying. It requires only a glance to determine the more or less acidifying or alkalizing nature of a meal, and of the meals suggested as healthy substitutes.

Keep in mind that the body needs foods that are naturally acidifying, such as proteins (dairy products, eggs, and so forth) and cereal grains, and that it is perfectly capable of neutralizing and eliminating their acids up to a certain point. A diet composed solely of alkaline foods is justified only if you are suffering from serious health problems brought on by acidification, and then only for a limited period. Otherwise, the diet can be gradually expanded to include more acidifying foods according to your physical ability to maintain a good acid–alkaline balance.

BREAKFAST

The three different breakfast menus provided here are among the most standard fare in contemporary culture. The replacement menus offered later in the chapter are merely suggestions or examples that can serve as guidelines. They can easily be changed and adapted according to individual need.

The conventional breakfast consists almost entirely of acidifying foods, except for butter, which is eaten in small quantity. What steps can be taken to make this meal more alkaline?

Replacing white bread with dark or whole-grain bread without yeast lowers the acidity level. The acid intake will be even less if the bread is replaced entirely by crackers or tortillas or chapatis prepared from whole-grain flour.

BREAKFAST: BREAD AND JAM

Alkalizing	Slightly acidifying	Very acidifying
EXAMPLE		
butter		white bread
		jam or jelly
		coffee or tea with milk
		and sugar
VARIATION 1		
butter	dark or whole-grain	
pear concentrate	bread	
coffee substitute,		
unsweetened or		
sweetened with		
natural sugar, or		
herb tea		
VARIATION 2		
butter	dark or whole-grain	
unsweetened coffee	bread	
substitute or herb	fromage blanc, cream	
tea, or fresh	cheese	
acidulated milk		

Jams and jellies are extremely acidifying for two reasons. First, the fruits used to make them are naturally acidic to varying degrees; and second, they typically have a very high sugar content (often as much as 50 percent).

Jelly and jam can be advantageously replaced by the pear or apple concentrates sold in health food stores. These are prepared from fruit juices that are filtered and reduced to solid form by water evaporation. They have the appearance and consistency of thin honey. These concentrates consist essentially of fructose. They have a very pleasant taste and retain a slight flavor of the fruit from which they were prepared. As they are intentionally made less acidic during the course of their preparation, they are truly alkalizing foods. Among similar products are spreads made from pears, apples, or other fruits. These are thicker and have not been deacidified, so they are less alkalizing than the concentrates, but they are much more alkaline than regular jams and jellies and therefore highly preferable.

Date concentrate is another similar alkaline product.

The conventional breakfast typically includes coffee, which is extremely acidifying because of its purine content (the same is true of black tea). As decaffeinated coffee is hardly any less acidifying, you should replace it entirely with one of the numerous substitute beverages made from chicory or roasted grains. As each of these has its own unique flavor, the best solution is to try them all until you find the one that tastes best to you. The aroma and flavor of these drinks aren't exactly like coffee, but because their color, consistency, and the way they are prepared and consumed are so similar to coffee, they make great substitutes that many inveterate coffee drinkers have turned to successfully.

Tea without theine is no more a solution than decaffeinated coffee. Green tea is less acidifying than black tea, but an even better option is herb teas. Mint and verbena are well known and very popular. Rosemary, sage, and thyme have stimulant properties that can partially replace those found in coffee and tea.

To sweeten herb teas or healthy coffee substitutes, it is better to use natural sugar obtained from the whole juice of the sugar cane or a sugar that is as unrefined as possible. Because it has not been refined, it still contains all the constituent elements of the juice (vitamins, enzymes, trace elements) and consequently can be metabolized easily by the body without producing acid waste products. White sugar, as well as "brown" sugar (which is simply white sugar that has had some of the molasses removed during the refining process added back in), should be strictly avoided.

Best of all would be not to use sugar of any kind. It is merely a matter of breaking the habit of sweetening your beverages, because these healthy substitutes taste delicious just as they are.

BREAKFAST: COFFEE AND PASTRY

Alkalizing	Slightly acidifying	Highly acidifying
EXAMPLE		
		coffee croissant, muffin, sweet roll
VARIATION 1		
herb tea or coffee substitute	whole-grain rusk bread (such as Melba toast) or other bread product	
VARIATION 2		
herb tea or coffee substitute dried fruits almonds		

Coffee and a Danish, croissant, or doughnut may be all you eat for breakfast if you are in a hurry or are not hungry in the morning. Such a meal may make you feel instantly energized, but the rush of energy has not been contributed by what you've just eaten. Rather, it has been borrowed from the body's own organic reserves by the alkaloids in the coffee. Foods that can truly provide energy are rich in glucides—fresh and dried fruits, cereal grains, and potatoes. Coffee contains no glucides, unless white sugar has been added. Pastry contributes some, but they are little in quantity and poor in quality.

Coffee's lack of contribution to physical vigor is not only due to the fact that it forces the body to convert the glucides and lipids stored in the tissues into glucose. This process, which is repeated with each cup of coffee or other stimulant, overtaxes the body and leads to the production of numerous acids. These acids then combine with those brought directly into the body by the coffee itself, and sometimes with those of the orange juice that has been taken for the benefit of its vitamin C content.

This double source of acidification engenders a state of chronic fatigue. Someone who regularly uses a stimulant like coffee quickly finds himself or herself in a vicious circle. To overcome fatigue, he or she takes more of the stimulant, which only maintains the state of debilitation.

A radical change is necessary to break this vicious circle. The solution involves giving the body genuine energetic assistance with a breakfast consisting of dark bread, butter, and pear concentrate, so that it can make the transition away from the artificial stimulation provided by coffee. The coffee is gradually—but in a short period of time—eliminated from the diet and replaced by naturally stimulating beverages such as herb teas with thyme, rosemary, and/or sage. Grain-based or chicory beverages can substitute for the taste and appearance of coffee without replicating its stimulant qualities.

The body obviously requires some time to get used to this new menu plan, but the rewards will greatly repay all the effort necessary to stick to it.

BREAKFAST: BIRCHER MUESLI

Alkalizing	Slightly acidifying	Very acidifying
EXAMPLE		
milk	breakfast cereal fresh fruit yogurt	
VARIATION 1		
milk (cow or soy)	crunchy flakes	
VARIATION 2		
cream cheese, fromage blanc dry fruit almonds	sweet, ripe fruit	

Cereal flakes are acidifying but need not be systematically eliminated from the diet, as they provide a good intake of energy for the body. Cereals are generally difficult to digest, and the poorer the digestion, the greater the problem of acidity. Untoasted or partially toasted flakes, such as are found in muesli or granola, are much harder to digest than those that have been baked or toasted to make them crunchy. In fact, the carbohydrates of cereal flakes are transformed into simpler substances by cooking. This acts as a kind of predigestion that makes digestion in the body easier. Crunchy and puffed cereals are therefore less acidifying.

There is one additional problem with cereals, and that is sugar. The sugar that is added to give a better flavor to the flakes is sometimes present in large quantity, which makes up for any reduction of the acidifying aspects by cooking. There are plenty of crunchy cereal blends, however, that have little or no sugar, or are sweetened with natural sugar or fruit juice rather than with refined white sugar.

To be digested properly, cereals need an alkaline digestive environment. Adding naturally acidic fresh fruits and/or yogurt to cereal upsets the digestion of the cereal and causes it to ferment, which engenders a number of acids and toxins. You can either eat cereals with milk, or eat fresh fruits with cream cheese, fromage blanc, or other soft, unripened cheeses, dried fruits, and almonds, all three of which are alkalizing.

Contrary to general belief, a blend of cereal flakes, fruits, and yogurt (or milk) does not conform to the famous muesli recipe created by Dr. Bircher.* His recipe used a single grain—rolled oats—in very modest helpings (one tablespoon per person), and he prescribed that the oats should be soaked overnight in water to predigest them. Although Dr. Bircher then added fresh fruits, this blend was much more digestible than the mixture known as muesli today.

---

*Dr. Maximilian Bircher (1867–1939) founded a health sanitorium in Zurich. He promoted a grain- and vegetable-based diet at a time when vegetables, fruits, and grains were considered foods for poor people.

Other Alkaline Breakfast Variations

Here are several additional suggestions for breakfast menus
that, while they may seem a little out of the ordinary, can be
quite helpful because of their alkaline character. Exclusively
consisting of alkaline foods, these meals are particularly recommended for those who need to follow a very strict alkaline
diet, but they are valuable for anyone simply as welcome variations on the daily meal.

OTHER BREAKFAST VARIATIONS

VARIATION 1	dried fruit
	almonds
	whey, buttermilk, or fresh white cheese
	herb tea or unsweetened coffee substitute
VARIATION 2	soaked dry fruits with soaking liquid
	fresh white cheese
	herb tea or unsweetened coffee substitute
VARIATION 3	mashed banana
	almonds or almond paste
	herb tea or unsweetened coffee substitute
VARIATION 4	chestnuts
	fresh white cheese
	herb tea or unsweetened coffee substitute
VARIATION 5	banana (or other sweet ripe fruit) smoothie made with cow's or soy or almond milk
VARIATION 6	raw carrots, raw fennel, etc.
	fresh white cheese
	unsweetened herb tea

MIDMORNING SNACK BREAK

Several hours—four to six normally—can elapse between breakfast and lunch. To last through an entire morning with the energy necessary to get work done or complete other activities, many people absolutely require the light boost that comes from a drink and perhaps a snack.

The most common refreshments today do fulfill this goal because they are rich in glucides, the preeminent energetic source. In most cases they are also acidifying, and therefore these snacks are not recommended if you are suffering from acid–alkaline imbalance. Below are some alternate suggestions.

MIDMORNING SNACK BREAK

Alkalizing	Slightly acidifying	Very acidifying
EXAMPLE		
		coffee with sugar cookies made with white flour and sugar, sometimes with chocolate
VARIATION 1		
coffee substitute sweetened with natural sugar	whole-grain cookies with little sugar	
VARIATION 2		
dried fruits almonds unsweetened herb tea		
VARIATION 3		
carrot juice		

Simply replacing pastry products or cookies made from white flour with those made from whole-grain flour, only slightly sweetened (ideally by raw cane sugar), reduces the acidifying effect of this kind of snack.

An alkaline beverage such as an herb tea or a healthy coffee substitute, which can be drunk either unsweetened or sweetened with natural sugar, should of course replace coffee (or black tea). You can also substitute crackers or cookies with dried fruits or almonds for the traditional pastry, and have an alkaline vegetable juice, such as carrot juice, for your beverage. A sensible choice of substitutes allows you to eat the kind of snack to which you are accustomed, but one with an entirely different effect on the body's acid–alkaline balance.

FRESH FRUIT SNACK

Alkalizing	Slightly acidifying	Very acidifying
	EXAMPLE	
		tart apple or other tart fruit
	VARIATION 1	
	sweet apple or other sweet, ripe fruit	
	VARIATION 2	
dried fruits unsweetened herb tea		
	VARIATION 3	
banana almonds		

Apples or other fruits are acidifying only if you have a deficiency in metabolizing acids. One option is to choose a sweet, ripe piece of fruit, which is less acidifying than less ripe, more tart fruit. There are two other options as well. The first is dried fruits—raisins, dates, bananas, and so forth— plus some almonds. The second is the only fruit that is absolutely alkaline: the banana. To be at its peak of flavor it must be completely ripe. A banana with some almonds is a delicious snack and a great alternative to the standard break-time fare.

SANDWICH AND SODA SNACK

Alkalizing	Slightly acidifying	Very acidifying
EXAMPLE		
		ham sandwich on white bread commercial soda or lemonade
VARIATION		
salad greens water	whole-grain bread cheese	

Commercial sodas and lemonades are very acidifying because of their high sugar content. From the dietary perspective these contain *bad sugar*; being highly refined, it enters the bloodstream rapidly and forces the pancreas to release insulin immediately to keep the blood sugar from rising too high (hyperglycemia). While this release may address the immediate crisis, the sudden and significant discharge of insulin generally causes the normal blood sugar level to drop too low, resulting in *hypo*glycemia and its consequent loss of energy. To restore the proper energy balance the body experiences a craving for sugar. If this need is satisfied again with a bad sugar, the resulting release of more insulin eventually exhausts the pancreas, and the body's internal environment becomes acidified due to the repeated intake of sugar. This in turn increases the body's demand for sugar, since the main symptom of acidification is fatigue. A vicious circle is created, similar to the one we examined with coffee. To get off this merry-go-round it is absolutely necessary to replace bad sugars (primarily white sugar and all the foods that contain it, such as soda, candy, pastry, etc.) with natural sugars: dried fruits, pear concentrate, granola bars.

Diet sodas with artificial sweeteners offer no alternative solution. Although they do not contain sugar, the ingredients normally used to replace sugar are by and large equally harmful.

Here are some more variations on the midmorning snack. The afternoon snacks outlined later in this chapter are also totally appropriate.

OTHER SNACK VARIATIONS

	Alkalizing	Slightly acidifying
VARIATION 1	cream cheese, large-curd cottage cheese, or other soft white cheese sweetened with pear concentrate or natural sugar	any sweet, fully ripe fruit
VARIATION 2	Granola bars not high in sugar, no chocolate	

	Alkalizing	Slightly acidifying
VARIATION 3	milk	crunchy cereal flakes
VARIATION 4	mashed banana almond paste	
VARIATION 5	almond milk	
VARIATION 6	vegetable juice	whole-grain cookies or crackers

Almond milk can be purchased in many health food stores; it can also be made by blending almond paste (available in health food stores) with a little water. This is a very flavorful, nutritious, and alkalizing beverage.

Vegetable juices (carrots, red beet, or vegetable juice cocktail) are a great source of energy because of the natural sugars they contain. Make sure the blends do not contain tomato, and that the method used to preserve them has not made them more acid (for example, lactofermentation). Keep this in mind especially if you are sensitive to acid.

LUNCH

The main meal of the day* most commonly consists of a protein (in the form of meat or fish), a starch (rice, pasta, or potatoes), and vegetables (green salad or a cooked side dish). This is normally followed by coffee and dessert, or, in some cases, cheese. How does such a meal rate on the scale of acid–alkaline balance?

---

*While some people enjoy the main meal of the day at noon, others eat this meal in the evening. The meal recommendations for lunch can be easily substituted for dinner, and vice-versa.

CLASSIC LUNCH MENU

Alkalizing	Slightly acidifying	Very acidifying
EXAMPLE		

cooked vegetables:
  carrots
green salad
		red meat
		sauce or gravy
		white rice
		strong cheese
		white bread
		wine or soda
		sweet dessert: custard,
		  pudding, cake,
		  cookies, ice cream
		coffee with sugar

VARIATION		

cooked vegetables:
  carrots
potatoes
green salad
unsweetened herb
  tea or water
	white meat
	whole-grain cookie
	  or cake sweetened
	  with natural sugar	

Meat and fish are acidifying foods. It is possible to reduce their acidifying effect by choosing white meats over red and lean fish over fish with high fat content. It would be sensible to replace the meat portion of the meal every other day with eggs or cheese, which satisfies the need for protein but in a less acidifying form. Note that the suggestion is to replace, not combine. Combining different proteins at one meal only complicates digestion and increases the acidification effect.

The fatty and flour-thickened sauces that often accompany meats have an acidifying effect; avoid them and choose grilled meat or fish instead.

Starchy foods made from grain (rice, pasta) are acidifying by nature, and even more so when refined, such as white rice or pasta made from white flour. Be careful not to overlook bread when you are analyzing this meal. Bread is acidifying, and people frequently eat quite a bit of it at lunch. Replacing bread with whole grains, such as brown rice or pasta made from whole wheat or other flours, can have a very salutary influence on the acid–alkaline balance. If this substitution does not have the desired results—as may be the case if you have a serious acidification problem—try replacing the grain-based foods with potatoes. When you are beginning a deacidification treatment, it is not really a hardship to eat potatoes on a daily basis if grain-based foods are too acidifying for your body. However, potatoes lose their alkalizing virtues if they are eaten as French fries, because the high fat content transforms them into acidifying foods.

In the lunch menus we have examined, the only truly alkalizing foods that can provide a counterbalance to the presence of acid foods are vegetables, raw or cooked. It is therefore very important to ensure that they represent a significant portion of the meal. When a piece of meat and the starch take up almost the entire surface of the plate, leaving room for only one or two spoonfuls of cooked vegetables, the role of the vegetables is no longer nutritious but merely decorative.

Sugary desserts have a double disadvantage: the additional acid intake provided directly by the sugar—most often white sugar—and the acids produced by the fermentation caused by the indigestible mixture of sugar and proteins. Cakes, pastries, custards, ice cream, and so forth are not recommended for this reason, and neither are natural fruits or fruit compotes. The ideal solution is to dispense with dessert altogether. If the urge for dessert is too strong to ignore, the best option is to limit it to simple foods: unflavored soft white cheese (cream cheese, fromage blanc), dry cookies with very little sugar, and so on.

The coffee that customarily brings the meal to a close stimulates the digestion to a slight degree, but because coffee is acidifying it is preferable to find a substitute, such as an herb tea made from nonacidifying and easily digested herbs: mint, verbena, balm, basil, rosemary, and so on.

PASTA MEALS

Alkalizing	Slightly acidifying	Very acidifying
EXAMPLE		
mixed tossed salad herbs	hot-pressed oil vinegar	spaghetti made from white flour tomato sauce Parmesan cheese
VARIATION		
mixed tossed salad virgin cold-pressed oil herbs	whole-grain pasta grated cheese, dash of vinegar or lemon juice, or yogurt	

Because of the numerous alkaline elements it contains, a generous helping of mixed salad (without tomatoes) can partially compensate for the acidifying nature of white pasta and tomato sauce. Tomatoes are well known as acidifying agents. When they are made into a sauce, their acidity increases because cooking both destroys their vitamin and mineral content and concentrates their acidic elements. When Parmesan cheese is added, the acidifying effect becomes even more intense; Parmesan is more acidic than many other cheeses, as you can tell by its taste.

Pasta-based meals can be alkalinized by using pasta made from whole-grain flour instead of refined white flour, and by eliminating the tomato sauce. Instead, eat pasta either with a little oil (virgin cold-pressed), or with some shredded cheese of a variety less acidic than Parmesan. If the idea of pasta without sauce is unthinkable, use a light white sauce or a pesto-type sauce.

It is important to keep the amount of vinegar (or lemon juice) in salad dressings small in proportion to the oil. Vinegar is highly acidic. Some people use more vinegar than oil in dressings, but many recipes call for a ratio of three parts oil to one part vinegar. The use of vinegar is so ingrained that many people find it hard to imagine a salad dressing without it. But you can create delicious salad dressings just with oil and herbs. Depending on your personal taste, soft white cheese, brewer's yeast, soy milk, vegetable juice, and so forth can also be used. The variations are endless.

If you still want a dressing that is slightly acidic, use vinegar or lemon juice, but in small doses.

The choice of oil is also important to minimize the acidifying effect of salad dressing. Choose high-quality virgin cold-pressed oil.

BEAN-BASED MEAL

Alkalizing	Slightly acidifying	Very acidifying
EXAMPLE		
cooked vegetables	tofu	lentils, soybeans, etc.
VARIATION 1		
cooked vegetables	whole grain tofu	
VARIATION 2		
cooked vegetables potatoes	tofu	

A bean-based dish using lentils, soybeans, or white beans, among many others, is common in vegetarian cooking. The bean dish is usually accompanied by a vegetable (and possibly a salad), but often it contains tofu (made from soybeans) or a grain as well (rice, couscous, corn, and so on). The purpose of these combinations is not simply gastronomic but nutritional. By themselves, neither grains nor beans contain all the essential amino acids the human body needs, but combined in the right proportions, grains and beans together form a complete protein.

Leguminous plants are extremely nutritious foods, but they are also very acidifying. They are hard to digest, especially when combined with cereal grains. Poor digestion creates more acids. Unfortunately, individuals who are unable to metabolize acids properly usually also have problems with their digestive systems in general. For them, the consumption of beans and other leguminous plant foods is double jeopardy. It would be far preferable for these individuals to eat beans only on an occasional basis (for example, well-cooked lentils), and to replace beans in their diet with cereals, which are just as nutritious but much, much easier to digest. People who are sensitive to acids should eat potatoes more often than grain-based dishes, because potatoes are easy to digest and always alkaline.

The menus above offer two more alkaline variations, one with the less acidifying cereals (corn, brown rice, spelt), and the other with potatoes. Vegetarians can obtain sufficient complete protein intake by supplementing these menus with tofu.

MEALS WITH WINE

Alkalizing	Slightly acidifying	Very acidifying
EXAMPLE		
cooked vegetables potatoes	lean fish	wine
VARIATION		
cooked vegetables potatoes water	lean fish	

Composed of equal amounts of alkalizing and acidifying foods, this meal seems relatively balanced. Nonetheless, it is not advised for people suffering from acidification or for those who have trouble metabolizing acids, because of the wine. Drunk as a regular accompaniment to meals, wine generally reduces digestive capability and represents a considerable intake of acids. The alcohol it contains is neutralized by the liver, but over a long period this work exhausts the organ. Furthermore, the tannins in wine lock up the mucous membranes of the digestive tract and reduce its ability to function properly. The weaknesses this causes have an effect on the body's ability to reduce the production of acids during the digestive process. As wine is acidifying by nature, it is better to drink it only on occasion, after your acid–alkaline balance has been restored, and never when you are experiencing any sort of health problem related to acids.

The meals listed below are basic meal templates. They can be infinitely varied by changing the raw and cooked vegetable, the cheese, and so on.

OTHER MEAL VARIATIONS

VARIATION 1	Raw vegetables with sprouts baked potatoes soft white cheese
VARIATION 2	cooked vegetables roasted potatoes soft white cheese
VARIATION 3	raw vegetables with almonds corn polenta soft white cheese
VARIATION 4	corn on the cob soft white cheese cooked vegetables
VARIATION 5	green salad cabbage chestnuts fresh acidulated milk
VARIATION 6	green salad/raw vegetables potatoes egg yolk (hard- or soft-boiled)

The following variations are not as alkalizing as the six just presented because they all contain one acidifying food. But this food item is only slightly acidifying and represents only a small portion of the total meal, so these variations can be considered as alkaline for all practical purposes.

LESS ALKALIZING MEAL VARIATIONS

	Alkalizing	Slightly acidifying
VARIATION 1	raw vegetables potatoes	Swiss-type cheese
VARIATION 2	green salad corn polenta	cheese or eggs
VARIATION 3	raw vegetables cooked vegetables chestnuts	cheese
VARIATION 4	green salad butter black olives soft white cheese	whole-grain crackers or dark bread
VARIATION 5	raw vegetables cooked vegetables soy sauce	fried brown rice (Oriental style)
VARIATION 6	green salad cooked vegetables	grain dish (spelt, etc.) or crepes or pasta
VARIATION 7	green salad potatoes	cheese or mushroom omelet
VARIATION 8	green salad tortilla with potatoes	eggs
VARIATION 9	mixed salad cooked vegetables	tofu

	Alkalizing	Slightly acidifying
VARIATION 10	green salad vegetables au gratin (with cream or milk) potatoes	cheese

MIDAFTERNOON SNACK OR TEA

Like the midmorning snack, the one in the afternoon supplies energy that bridges the gap between the previous meal and dinner. As the greatest part of the day is now past, especially that part of the day that makes up most professional activities, a natural sense of fatigue begins to make its presence felt. The reason for this is that the energy supplied by the foods eaten at lunch has been significantly depleted. Blood sugar levels are therefore low, and the need for glucides is making itself felt, often powerfully, which can drive a person to consume foods that are unhealthy and acidifying.

Sweets such as candy bars or pastries are characterized by their high refined-sugar content and usually by high levels of unhealthy fats. These products cause blood sugar levels to rise rapidly and give the body a boost with a quick supply of energy. But as we have already explained, refined sugar is one of the biggest culprits in acidification of the body.

SWEET SNACK

Alkalinizing	Slightly acidifying	Very acidifying
EXAMPLE		
		chocolate candy
VARIATION		
dried fruit: dates, figs		

A good replacement for a candy bar or pastry is dried fruit. The high natural sugar content and strong flavor make dried fruits feel filling, and the natural sugars do not trigger a hypoglycemic episode. There is a wide variety of dried fruits to choose from with many different flavors and textures, so everyone should be able to find something to his or her taste.

The chart below examines pastries, which are composed of white flour, saturated fats, and refined sugars, three ingredients that are highly acidifying. When this snack is washed down with coffee, black tea, or soda, the acidifying effects are increased.

By replacing a pastry with a whole-grain muffin sweetened with natural sugar, dried fruits, or pear concentrate, and replacing soda, coffee, or black tea with herb tea, you can lessen the acidifying effect considerably.

Pastries can also be replaced by any of a number of commercially manufactured whole-grain cookies available in the supermarket, or any other of the alkaline variations suggested in the chart. Sodas or caffeinated beverages can easily be eliminated in favor of smoothies or fruit smoothies.

PASTRY SNACK

Alkalizing	Slightly acidifying	Very acidifying
	EXAMPLE	
		pastry, black tea or soda
	VARIATION 1	
herb tea	whole-grain cake or cookies with natural sugar	
	VARIATION 2	
banana smoothie	smoothie with sweet, ripe fruit	

Fruit smoothies are not only extremely energizing thanks to their constituent fruits, but they also provide energy over a long period. The glucide (fruit)–protein (milk) blend stabilizes blood sugar levels because the proteins diminish the speed with which the body burns off the glucides and thus also acts as a brake against hypoglycemia. Smoothies can be made from regular milk or from cream cheese thinned with a little water. Soy milk can also be used. To make a smoothie, simply put the fruits and liquid in a blender and blend until smooth. If necessary, you can add a natural sweetener to taste.

The classic snack of bread with butter and/or jelly with cocoa or chocolate milk can be transformed from an acidifying meal into a more alkalizing one simply by a more judicious selection of its components. By choosing dark or whole-grain bread over white, substituting a natural sweetener like pear concentrate for jelly, and replacing the cocoa or chocolate milk with herb tea or plain milk, you have changed this snack into a completely alkalizing meal.

BREAD AND JAM SNACK

Alkalizing	Slightly acidifying	Very acidifying
EXAMPLE		
butter		white bread
		jam or jelly
		hot chocolate
		or chocolate milk
VARIATION		
butter	dark or whole-grain	
pear concentrate	bread	
herb tea or milk		

Fruits and fruit juices do not have the same acidifying effects on everyone. They have been classified among the acidifying foods because this book is primarily directed toward people whose metabolisms are deficient in dealing with acids. For these individuals, yogurt, which is naturally acid, can be replaced by soft white cheese or fresh acidophilus milk, and fresh fruits by dried fruits such as bananas or raisins, which, if they have been soaked beforehand, go better with the soft white cheese.

FRUIT SNACK*

Alkalizing	Slightly acidifying	Very acidifying
	EXAMPLE	
	sweet, ripe fruit fresh yogurt	tart fruit or fruit juice aged yogurt
	VARIATION	
dried fruit soft white cheese		

*A midafternoon snack serves exactly the same purpose as a midmorning snack, so these meals are easily interchangeable. Any alkaline variation suggested for the midmorning snack would work just as well here.

EVENING MEAL

Dinner for some people is the big meal of the day and uses the same types of menus as the standard lunch meals we examined earlier. For other people, dinner is a much smaller affair. Despite its straightforward appearance, it is often much more complicated and much more acidifying than you might think. This is especially true for the evening meal composed of bread, butter and jelly or cold cuts and cheese, and coffee—a repast that is common because it requires little preparation.

We now understand the acidifying nature of coffee, bread, and jelly. Cold cuts and cheese as high-protein foods are also highly acidifying, but cold cuts are much more so because of their greater concentration of saturated fats. On the digestive level, it is not so simple, and it is even more complex on the level of acid–alkaline balance. In fact, when a meal of this kind is composed totally of acidifying foods, the body is forced to neutralize the acids it ingests solely with the alkaline substances it draws from its own tissues.

To restore balance to this kind of meal, include a generous helping of green salad or raw vegetables. Rather than drink coffee, pick another beverage such as herb tea; or, best of all, vegetable soup, which is rich in alkaline substances. By replacing white bread with whole-wheat or other whole-grain bread and strong cheese with milder cheese, you can lower the acid levels of this kind of meal even further.

LIGHT SUPPER OR LUNCH

Alkalizing	Slightly acidifying	Very acidifying
EXAMPLE		
butter	cheese honey	white bread cold cuts strong cheese jam or jelly coffee
VARIATION		

green vegetables
  or raw vegetables
  or vegetable soup
herb tea
	whole-grain bread
	or crackers
	 cheese
	honey	

Pies and fruit tarts are acidifying because of their combination of ingredients. The fruits used for making pies are often unripe and call for additional sugar. Furthermore, the combination of starch (pastry crust) and an acid food (fruits) upsets the digestion and allows fermentation to occur, encouraging the production of acids.

There are no good alternatives to fruit tarts or pies. If you are suffering from acidification and crave such foods, you should simply be aware of their nature and consequences and limit their intake. However, a less acidic variation can be made from unrefined flour, a natural sugar, and fully ripened fruits.

FRUIT PIES AND TARTS

Alkalizing	Slightly acidifying	Very acidifying
	EXAMPLE	
		pastry crust fruits white sugar
	VARIATION	
	pastry crust from unrefined flour natural sugar fully ripened fruits	

Pizza is an extremely acidifying food because of its principal ingredients. Two alternatives are possible, but neither includes tomatoes, which are always acidifying. The first is a vegetable pie. The acidification effects can be made less significant by the vegetables and a crust made from unrefined, whole-grain flour. The second alternative is a cheese pizza. It is not truly an alkalizing food, but its slightly acidifying nature can be diminished even further if it is accompanied by a large green salad or a generous helping of raw vegetables.

PIZZA

Alkalizing	Slightly acidifying	Very acidifying
	EXAMPLE	
mozzarella cheese black olives	whole-grain pizza crust grated cheese	white flour pizza crust tomatoes or tomato sauce
	VARIATION 1	
pizza with vegetable toppings	whole-grain pizza crust grated cheese	
	VARIATION 2	
green salad	pizza with cheese whole-grain pizza crust grated cheese	

In addition to the other alkaline variations that were already listed as lunch suggestions, vegetable soup is another evening meal possibility.

Vegetable soup offers a countless number of possibilities for varied meals. With a simple change of ingredients you can create a limitless range of soups that look and taste entirely different from one another. Be careful, however, not to thicken soups with cereal-based starches; use potatoes instead. When accompanied by a little cheese (to provide protein) and possibly some whole-grain bread, soup is a very pleasant meal, especially during the cold months of the year.

Part Three

NEUTRALIZING AND ELIMINATING ACIDS

6

Alkaline Supplements

$$\sim\!\!\sim$$

While the adoption of an alkaline diet can interrupt the acid-ification process and reduce the concentration of acids in the body, diet alone is not sufficient to completely remove excess acids from the body's internal environment. The reformed diet needs the reinforcement of alkaline supplements.

The greatest problem for people suffering from acidification is not the presence of acids circulating on the surface—in the bloodstream, for example—but the concentrated mass of acids that have accumulated in the deep inner tissues. *How did these acids get there in the first place?*

Blood does not contain great amounts of acid. Because the pH of blood must stay within a narrow range, the body seeks to remove acids from the bloodstream as rapidly as possible.

In addition to the neutralization of acids by the body's buffer system, the body has two other means for disposing of them. The first, which is also the most beneficial, is the elimination of acids through urine and sweat, which keeps the acids from dangerously altering the healthy pH level of the blood.

Unfortunately, the quantities of acids that have built up

are often beyond the ability of the skin and kidneys to deal with effectively. The body is then forced to use a second option to protect the integrity of the blood pH. This consists of directing the acids not to the organs of elimination, which would discharge them, but into the tissues, which can withstand fluctuations of pH levels better than the blood. For people whose lifestyle and diet are highly acidifying, and for those who are metabolically deficient in dealing with acids, this repression process is constant. As each new ingestion of acids forces the previous acids a little deeper into the tissues, the amount of acids that build up can be considerable.

The deacidification of the body, or the correction of an acidified internal environment, therefore requires the neutralization and elimination of a very large quantity of acids. It might seem that an intensive, sustained period of cleansing would allow all this built-up acid to be eliminated by stimulating the skin and kidneys to free the body of these toxins. Unfortunately, this is not the case.

To reach the skin and kidneys, the acids embedded in the tissues must first enter the bloodstream, which then carries them to the renal and subcutaneous filtering systems. This is where the difficulty lies, as the blood cannot take in much acid at one time without risking too great a deviation from its normal pH level, endangering the smooth operation and even the survival of the entire body.

The blood, therefore, accepts only minimal quantities of acid at a time and prevents any excess from entering, which strongly reduces the possibility of eliminating the acids through the skin and kidneys. To address this situation, the acids can be made to enter the blood in an altered form that causes them to lose their acid characteristics. This form is that of a *neutral salt,* which is obtained by the addition of an alkaline substance. An acid and alkaline combined form a neutral salt.

To neutralize each acid you want removed from the body you need a corresponding alkaline substance, but the elimination routes do not supply such substances. Alkalines brought in by an alkaline diet, even a strict one, are often not enough to do the job or would require far too much time (years) to perform it efficiently. The change in diet is primarily meant to deal with the body's current need for alkaline substances, not for disposing of the previous accumulation of acids. It is therefore imperative to provide alkaline substances in addition to those the body is ingesting through food. This is possible with alkaline supplements, preparations containing the principal alkaline minerals—calcium, potassium, magnesium, and so forth—in a form that is easily assimilated by the body.

Taking these alkaline supplements on a regular basis supports the body's efforts and greatly accelerates the process of deacidification. The supplements also provide quicker relief to the patient experiencing the painful symptoms or harmful disorders caused by excess acids in the body. Thanks to supplements, these disorders diminish, often in a remarkably short period.

The disappearance of symptoms and superficial disorders does not mean that the body has gotten rid of all its acids. They still remain in the deeper tissue layers, but the reduction in their concentration causes an initial disappearance of the minor problems that their presence may cause. Later, if this kind of supplemental therapy is maintained for a sufficient period, the internal environment is cleansed of all the acids that have built up and is therefore able to return to its normal functioning. The state of total health reached in this way can then be maintained without taking alkaline supplements but simply by adopting the appropriate lifestyle and following an adequate diet.

There are more than a dozen different kinds of alkaline supplements available today, whereas twenty years ago there were only three or four. This increase is due to the growing public awareness of the health problems caused by acid–alkaline imbalance.

This diversity offers a great advantage because, although the supplements are all fundamentally similar, their differences and individual features allow their use to be adapted to the widely varying needs of a greater number of individuals.

The following analysis focuses on twelve products. It is by no means exhaustive, but examines supplements with which the author has personal experience. Names of distributors of these and similar products available in the United States are provided in the Resources section. All these products are of proven effectiveness. They are listed not in order of effectiveness or preference but alphabetically. If readers know of alkaline supplements that are not mentioned here, they can easily evaluate them using the criteria outlined later in the chapter.

The twelve products are Alcabase, Alkala, Basin, Basinette, Equilibre-Vital, Erbasit, Flügge's Alkaline Blend, Megabase, Nimbasit, Rebasit, Sanarter Basic, and Somona Nutritious Alkaline Salts. (For information on where to obtain Equilibre-Vital, Erbasit, Megabase, and Nimbasit, please see the Resources section at the end of this book.)

In the section that follows, we look at the composition of

these alkaline supplements, how much of them to take and when (dosage), and the length of time they should be taken (see the summary chart on page 132).

COMPOSITION OF ALKALINE SUPPLEMENTS

The majority of these preparations contain five alkaline minerals: calcium, potassium, magnesium, iron, and manganese. To make a supplement with only one of these minerals would be a mistake, because the body's needs are well defined, and too large a dose of any mineral can surpass the body's capacity to assimilate it. Furthermore, the body's buffer system makes use of all these minerals, each of which has a specific reason to be included in these combinations.

The Five Base Minerals

Calcium (Ca) is the mineral with the greatest presence in the human body. It is found mainly in the skeleton, but it is an indispensable part of many of the other tissues, primarily those that make up the nervous system. Potassium (K) plays a fundamental role in cellular exchanges. If there is a deficiency of this mineral the body's energy production is poor, and muscle cramps occur. Magnesium (Mg) is well known for its calming effect on the nervous sytem and its stimulating effect on the immune system. Iron (Fe) is necessary to carry oxygen in the blood, which is of critical importance for people who have trouble metabolizing acids, since, among other deficiencies, they cannot oxidize volatile acids properly. Manganese (Mn) acts as a catalyst in numerous biochemical reactions.

If these minerals are to be of optimum benefit, it is very important that the proportion of each one in the combination is carefully chosen. In fact, the use of different nutrients by the body depends on the subtle balances between these minerals. For example, too high a presence of one can act like a brake on the assimilation of another, or the lack of one may prevent a second from being used, even if it is available in large quantity.

There are some slight variations in the ingredients of the different alkaline supplements described here, but all are balanced. However, some do not contain all five of the minerals listed (for example, the Alkala preparation does not contain iron, magnesium, or manganese; the Flügge base blend does not contain either potassium or iron; and the Megabase blend is missing both manganese and iron). Blends of this nature should be chosen when for one reason or another you need to restrict intake of one or more of these minerals.

Presence or Absence of Sodium (Na)

Sodium is a mineral used in great quantities by most people on a daily basis, as it is found in ordinary salt in the form of sodium chloride. The principal property of salt is the retention of water in the tissues. One gram of salt will retain 11 grams of fluid.

Consequently, excess sodium results in general or local edema (such as swollen ankles or fingers). When the tissues are swollen, blood pressure can rise dangerously high (hypertension) and put strain on the heart, causing it to tire. The kidneys may also deteriorate prematurely from overwork, because they are responsible for eliminating sodium excess.

An excess of sodium in the tissues can be corrected by either reducing the intake of salt or by increasing intake of potassium, which is the antagonist of sodium.

While excessive sodium in the body has a tendency to raise blood pressure and is generally stimulating, a sodium deficiency results in hypotension and apathy.

Among the alkaline supplements listed, two do not contain sodium, Sanarter Basic and Somona. Although equally effective when it comes to neutralizing acids, these blends are especially recommended for individuals who want to deacidify but who also suffer from water retention, edema, or heart or kidney problems.

On the other end of the spectrum, the Rebasit preparation has a very high sodium content (74 percent), which makes it unsuitable for anyone suffering from the problems just mentioned. It is, however, recommended for people with low blood pressure or who lack vitality and muscle tonicity. All the other supplements listed contain modest quantities of sodium, which, furthermore, are always combined with its antagonist, potassium.

Silica

Silica is an acid mineral, as it appears in the form of silicic acid. Its presence in alkaline supplements is easily explained. Silica is of great help in a large number of the disorders that affect acidified people, including hair loss, fragile nails, dental cavities, skin problems, and joint pains. The soundness of the skeletal frame, teeth, nails, and hair, as well as the suppleness of the skin, depend in large part on silica.

Seven of the alkaline blends listed contain this important mineral: Alkala, Erbasit, Flügge, Megabase, Rebasit, Sanarter Basic, and Somona. Silica does not have an acidifying effect when ingested in these preparations because it is present in very small quantities, whose acidity is neutralized by the large amounts of alkaline substances with which it is combined. Its benefits can thus be obtained without causing more acidification.

This is not the case with the silica found in horsetail and millet, which are often recommended for combatting disorders caused by mineral depletion, because their content of this mineral is much higher than the content of the alkaline supplement blends.

Other Minerals

Several minerals (copper, strontium, and vanadium) are used in the preparation of the supplement Basin, but not in any other. These minerals do not play a major role in the body's buffer system, but they can contribute to restoring the acid–alkaline balance because of their specific properties. Copper, for example, is essential for forming red corpuscles, so it is important in the transport of oxygen and the acids dependent upon it. The roles played by strontium and vanadium are not clear.

Form of the Supplements

The minerals contained in these alkaline supplements must be in a form the body can metabolize properly. In the blends listed they are most often prepared as salts, meaning combinations of an acid and a base. But the acids used for this purpose are weak and easily oxidized, so the body can get rid of them quickly, leaving the alkaline substance behind. The majority of blends consist of citrates—alkaline salts with a weak acid component—whose acidic portion is easily oxidized and expelled from the body by the lungs. Other forms of alkaline mineral blends are carbonates, tartrates, sulfates, gluconates, and lactates.

Preparations containing weak acids can show an acid pH reading on litmus paper. This in no way means that the these products have an acidifying effect, because the acid portion of the salts absorbed by the body is rapidly eliminated, even by people who have a metabolic deficiency in handling acids.

Whey

Whey is well known for its cleansing qualities. It stimulates renal elimination (diuretic effect), intestinal elimination (laxative effect), and elimination by the liver. It therefore encourages the elimination of toxins in general, including acids.

Whey is also rich in minerals, most of them alkaline, which makes it an excellent source for restoring minerals to the body—potassium in particular, as whey is exceptionally rich in this substance (2 percent).

When combined with alkaline blends, whey is therefore doubly useful, as it encourages elimination and restores mineral content to the body. Four products contain whey: Basinette, Nimbasit, Sanarter Basic, and Somona Salts.

People who are allergic to milk sugar or who are lactose intolerant should not take products containing whey.

Medicinal Plants

Plants with medicinal properties have also been added to certain blends. Nettle, which encourages the production of red corpuscles, is anti-anemic (Basinette, Nimbasit). Anise and wormwood, like wood charcoal, stimulate the digestive processes and fight intestinal fermentation (Megabase). Erbasit contains elder, linden, fennel, chamomile, and marigold, plants that have beneficial effects on both digestion and elimination, providing additional support to the deacidification process.

COMPOSITION, TASTE, AND APPEARANCE OF ALKALINE SUPPLEMENTS

Product	Ca	K	Mg	Fe	Mn	Na	Si	Others	Whey	Medicinal plants	Taste	Powder	Tablets
Alcabase	•	•	•	•	•	•					salty or lemony	•	•
Alkala	•	•	•	•	•	•					salty	•	
Basin	•	•	•	•	•	•		Cu,Va,St			salty	•	
Basinette	•	•	•	•	•	•		yeast	•	nettles	cherry		•
Equilibre-vital	•	•	•	•	•	•					broth	•	•
Erbasit	•	•	•		•	•	•			elder	orange	•	•
Flügge	•	•	•	•	•	•	•				salty	•	
Megabase	•	•	•	•	•	•	•			anise, absinthe, wood charcoal	anise	•	
Nimbasit	•	•	•	•	•	•	•		•	nettles	salty		•
Rebasit	•	•	•	•	•	•					salty	•	
Sanarter Basic	•	•	•	•	•		•		•		orange		•
Somona	•	•	•	•	•	•	•		•		orange	•	

Other Additives

Other natural substances in these alkaline mineral blends, such as malt or dextrin, are used simply as a binding agent and have negligible effects on health. One exception is the natural brewer's yeast, an energy booster, in the combination Basinette.

Taste

The taste of alkaline supplements is important. A therapy using one of these supplements can last for months. Persevering and sticking to a regular schedule are much easier if the taste of the product is agreeable.

Some of these preparations have a neutral flavor with a more or less salty accent from the different salts used in their manufacture (Alcabase, Alkala, Basin, Flügge, Nimbasit, Rebasit). Some products are flavored with fruit pulp. Alcabase has a lemony taste, Basinette is cherry flavored, and Erbasit, Sanarter Basic, and Somona are flavored with orange. The Megabase product has an anise flavor, but the most distinctive flavor is that of Equilibre-Vital, which tastes like broth.

Alkaline supplements are available in powdered form, to be blended with water, or in tablet form, to be swallowed with a glass of water.

ALKALINE SUPPLEMENT INTOLERANCE

Except for the warning given earlier about preparations containing large quantities of sodium, generally speaking alkaline supplements are very easily tolerated. They can on occasion cause intestinal gas and mild diarrhea at the beginning of a treatment. Most often this is not due to an intolerance for these substances, but is a temporary manifestation of taking too much initially before the body has had time to adjust.

The solution to this problem is to start with small doses and gradually increase the quantity being taken. If discomfort persists, it is probably because an ingredient in the blend is not suitable for the individual in question. In that case, a different blend should set everything right.

ALKALINE SUPPLEMENT DOSAGES

In contrast to most remedies, alkaline supplements have no fixed dosage instructions. The dosage always depends on the individual, so you are responsible for figuring out which dose is correct for your needs.

To determine the right dosage, it is of fundamental importance to take as much of an alkaline supplement as necessary to obtain a urinary pH reading that falls between 7 and 7.5.

Because many people are unaware of or ignore this rule of thumb, they do not gain maximum benefit from this therapy. The reason for taking alkaline supplements is to supply the body with its daily alkaline requirements so as to neutralize the acids that saturate its tissues. Of course, this quantity varies from one person to the next, just as the degree of acidification is not the same for everyone.

When the dosage is too low to meet the body's needs, neutralization of acids still occurs, but to a much smaller degree than could have been achieved, so the treatment does not live up to expectations. The treatment also takes much longer and is never complete, because the body still lacks enough alkaline substance to detoxify the deep tissues of their acids.

The purpose of alkaline supplement–based therapies is to neutralize and eliminate not only surface acids, but also those that have built up in the depths of the body's internal environment, until they have all been removed and optimum health has been restored. It is only at this point that the body is completely detoxified of acid wastes. This is a real cure, not simply superficial improvement of symptoms. In fact, the true nature of the condition is not its surface symptoms but the toxic state of the body's internal environment when saturated with acid wastes.

To determine the appropriate individual dosage levels of the alkaline supplement you have chosen, first take a series of urinary pH readings to determine the average value. For four to five days, measure urinary pH with the litmus paper and record the results on a suitable chart (see the sample on page 28 and the "Urinary pH Record" chart on page 164). This should be long enough to allow a clear indication of your average pH. To see the effect of the supplement, continue taking the urinary pH as you begin the treatment.

For example, let's say you have a urinary pH that is more or less 5 throughout the day. A pH reading of 5 is acid, even highly acid, a sign of an acidified internal environment. To detoxify this acidic state, an alkaline supplement is definitely called for. To determine the ideal dosage, begin with small doses and gradually increase them until the urinary pH reaches 7 to 7.5.

Start with a level teaspoon of powder mixed with water and take it before each of the three main meals of the day. If the urinary pH rises to 6, increase the next day's dosage to a heaping rather than a level teaspoonful of powder three times a day. If this increase results in a pH of 7 to 7.5, you can maintain this dosage for the duration of the therapy. If the urinary pH remains below 7, you need to increase the dosage further—to two heaping teaspoonfuls before each meal, or even three.

Do not worry about taking too much. If you have to take a significant amount to bring the urinary pH to 7 to 7.5, it is because your body needs it.

Once you have determined the proper dosage for the duration of the therapy by this means, there is no longer any need to take daily readings of urinary pH.

People suffering from acidification whose urine is alkaline cannot use urinary pH readings as a basis for determining the proper dosages of alkaline supplements. They should start with an average dose and try to guide themselves according to whether their symptoms get better or worse.

MONTHLY MONITORING

As the therapy progresses, the acids that have built up in the body are neutralized and eliminated. As their concentration gradually diminishes, so too does the body's need for alkaline products to neutralize them. After a certain period the dosage that was necessary at the beginning of the therapy may be too high for the body's new requirements.

Therefore, once-a-month readings of urinary pH should be taken over a one- to two-day period. As long as the pH remains between 7 and 7.5, continue taking the supplement at its current dosage. If the reading is below 7—if it is 6.5 or lower—increase the dosage. This is rarely necessary, however. More often than not, after several weeks or months (some treatments may require a year or two) the pH climbs to 8 or higher. This means the body no longer requires as much alkaline material as before and is getting rid of the excess in the urine, which naturally becomes more alkaline. At this point you can reduce the dosage until the urinary pH again reads between 7 and 7.5. In this way the body receives exactly what it requires to correct its internal environment.

This kind of dosage readjustment should be performed on a regular basis over the course of the therapy. In this way, the quantity of the alkaline supplements in the diet will gradually diminish.

LENGTH OF TREATMENT

Alkaline supplement therapies are undertaken for as long as the body needs them to clear up the acid toxification of its internal environment. This varies from one individual to the next. It can last anywhere from six months to two years, based on the degree of acidification. This may seem like a long time, but it is quite short when you consider that the body was building up these acid waste deposits for a good number of years before any health problems appeared.

The sign that the therapy has reached its goal and can now be stopped is when you have a urinary pH of 7 to 7.5 without taking any alkaline supplements. This value appears naturally because the further the treatment progresses, the greater the reduction in the need for alkaline supplements. One day, following the monthly pH reading, the small amount of alkaline supplements you are still taking can be eliminated.

Of course, it is only the alkaline supplement–based therapy that you stop, not the alkaline diet that you have been following in parallel. You must maintain the diet to conserve all you have gained with the therapy. If you abandon the diet, acidification of the body picks up anew, and all your old health problems reappear.

The strictness of this alkaline diet depends on the physical capacities of each individual to metabolize acids properly. It remains quite strict for those who have trouble metabolizing acids, but most people have much greater leeway. In all cases the soundness of the diet can be determined through urinary pH. If it becomes acid again, the diet has become too expansive.

At the end of an alkaline supplement treatment the body is thoroughly cleansed of acid wastes. This is reflected by a long-forgotten state of vitality and well-being. Many people have said they never realized how good one could feel when one is healthy!

If your ability to metabolize acids properly is poor, the diet necessary to maintain a urinary pH of 7 to 7.5 would be so strict that not only would it be impossible to follow but it would probably create other deficiencies. In fact, the intake of proteins and grains would be so limited that the body could not obtain all the nutrients it needs.

If you have this particular metabolic deficiency, you should not attempt to follow a diet that is perfect in theory but unrealizable in practice. Instead, include a degree of variety in your diet and compensate for any excess acids by continuing to take alkaline supplements. Under certain circumstances, this is the only means of dealing with the physical deficiency while maintaining a diet and lifestyle that are physiologically and psychologically acceptable.

7

Draining Acids

ॐ

Up to now, the main topic of this book has been how to reduce excessive intake of acids through adequate diet and alkaline supplements.

However, there are two causes for acidification of the body's internal environment. One is the ingestion of excessive amounts of acids; the other is their insufficient elimination. This chapter examines how to stimulate the organs responsible for elimination so they can get rid of as much acid as possible.

The organs responsible for the elimination of acids are the kidneys and skin, on the one hand, and the lungs on the other. It is important to make a distinction between these two groups of organs of elimination, because they each deal with different kinds of acids. The skin and kidneys eliminate strong acids, such as uric acid, sulfuric acid, and phosphoric acid—the acids that primarily come from animal proteins. The lungs eliminate the weak or volatile acids, such as citric acid, pyruvic acid, oxalic acid, and so forth, that derive from plants in the form of carbon dioxide (CO_2).

ACID DRAINAGE THROUGH THE KIDNEYS

Although they can eliminate weak acids, the kidneys specialize in the treatment of strong acids. This elimination is limited in quantity, because it is a relatively difficult task requiring a complex set of procedures. First the wastes have to be filtered out of the blood. Next they are diluted in fluid so they do not cause injury to the mucous membranes of the urinary system. They are then conducted to the bladder, where they are stored until they are expelled from the body by urination.

The quantity of acids that the kidneys eliminate each day may not match the quantity of acids consumed and produced by the body on that day. Dietary reform that reduces the intake of acids helps, but it is also important to stimulate the kidneys to increase the amounts of acids they filter and void, especially for people whose kidneys operate below their actual capacity. This is not a matter of kidney disease but rather of an insufficiency or renal laziness.

A primary means of stimulating the work of the kidneys is to increase the amount of liquids you consume. A major aspect of the renal filtration process is the difference between the blood pressure that pushes into the renal filter and the opposing resistance of this filter. If the blood pressure is greater than that of the filter, the blood is pushed through the filter and its acids removed. In the opposite case, the filtration works poorly because the lack of pressure is a hindrance. By drinking more than usual you can increase your blood volume, which then exerts greater pressure. The inevitable result is more copious urination.

The role played by pressure in urination explains why coffee—which raises blood pressure—increases urination, and also why fear stimulates the need to urinate (adrenaline secretion raises blood pressure).

An effective way of drinking enough liquid over the course of the day—and an easy way to remember to do so—is to systematically have a drink after each time you urinate. Urination is prompted by an amount of liquid in the body over a certain tolerance threshold. Voiding this liquid through urination reduces the amount of liquid until it is beneath the threshold of tolerance, and it remains below this threshold as long as no new liquid has been drunk. Taking a drink immediately following urination, in a quantity equal to or greater than what was eliminated, causes the liquid level of the body to rise above the tolerance threshold again, and this triggers a new elimination cycle automatically.

The volume of liquid that thus travels through the body encourages the elimination of toxins, because it can easily dilute and transport numerous acids and salts without causing the urine to become overly concentrated. The bed of a stream is much cleaner if large quantities of water flow through it as opposed to a small sluggish current.

Medicinal Plants for Draining Acids

While an abundant supply of liquid encourages elimination, it is also possible to increase the quantities of acids eliminated from the body by stimulating the kidneys' filtration capacities with diuretic (urination producing) medicinal plants. These plants and herbs allow the kidneys to handle much larger quantities of toxins, and the body is therefore able to get rid of those toxins much more quickly.

Through the action of these plants the renal filter first gets rid of the wastes that are burdening it. Once this has been accomplished, it cleanses the blood of any acids it is holding, allowing those just outside the blood capillaries—the acids embedded a little deeper in the tissues—to enter the circulatory system and be transported to the kidneys. Once these acids have been eliminated, those embedded even deeper in the tissues enter the circulatory system for eventual removal. Such an elimination process reaches progressively deeper tissues until, finally, the body's entire internal environment is cleansed.

To be really effective diuretic plants must be taken in the proper dosages; people usually do not take enough, and so have minimal or no results. With the correct dosages the effects are unmistakable. As the urine becomes more heavily charged with acids it takes on a darker color, and the odor becomes stronger. The frequency of urination increases, as does the quantity of urine eliminated.

To determine the optimum dosage, you need to increase the average doses suggested until you obtain the desired effects. Diuretic plant medicines should be taken three times daily at least—morning, noon, and in the evening before supper. This ensures that the kidneys can depend on their support for the entire day. These therapies should last anywhere from four to six weeks and be renewed after a break of a week or two for a total of two to three rounds. It is also a good idea to vary the plants used from one therapeutic session to another, as the body has a tendency to become accustomed to any given plant and stops reacting as strongly to the stimulus the plant provides after a certain period.

As with foods, some of these plants (primarily horsetail—rich in silicic acid—and birch) also contain acids and thus should not be taken by people with metabolic-acid deficiencies.

When prepared as teas diuretic plants enter the body in liquid form, thus intensifying their effect. However, preparing them this way does take a little time, and not everyone enjoys drinking these teas. Fortunately most plants are also available in tablet form and as tinctures, both equally valid alternatives. These forms are also more practical for when you are traveling or eating out at a restaurant. The list below defines the various means of preparing plant medicines.

PLANT MEDICINE PREPARATIONS

Tea or infusion: A drink obtained by steeping a plant or herb in hot water for several minutes.

Decoction: A beverage obtained by boiling plant material in water in a tightly sealed pot.

Tinctures (drops): A solution of a plant's active principles in an alcohol base.

Tablets: Medicinal plants are dried, crushed into a powder, and compacted into tablet form.

Tisane: A mixture of different plants prepared as a tea.

Many plants are available to assist the kidneys in draining acids from the body. The list below gives several recommendations for plant therapies and the best method of preparation. In these recipes a cup refers to the standard six-ounce teacup.

PLANT MEDICINES FOR KIDNEY STIMULATION

- Black currant: The leaves have a diuretic quality and make a very pleasant-tasting beverage. Make a tea by mixing 1 handful of leaves (1$^1/_2$ oz; 40 g) per quart of water, or 1 tablespoon per cup. Steep at least 10 minutes. Drink 3 cups daily before or between meals.

- Artichoke: The leaves (not the bracts of the flowers) have an excellent diuretic effect. They also stimulate liver function. Artichoke leaves make a bitter-tasting drink. Mix $1/3$ oz (10 g) of leaves per quart of water, or 1 teaspoonful per cup. Steep for 10 minutes. Drink 3 cups a day before meals.

- Cherry stems: The peduncles or stems are used for their diuretic action. Save the stems when you eat cherries and put them aside to dry. This makes a very refreshing beverage. Mix 1 handful of stems per quart of water. Make a decoction by boiling for 10 minutes. Drink 3 cups a day at a minimum.

- Linden bark: Linden bark is an excellent means for draining acids from the body (also recommended for all forms of rheumatism, kidney stones, and gallstones). Make a decoction by mixing $1^1/2$ oz (40 g) of bark per quart of water. Boil until the liquid is reduced to $1/4$ of the volume. Drink the decoction during the day. Traditional therapy calls for this beverage to be drunk 20 days a month for several months.

- Pilosella: An excellent diuretic and disinfectant for the urinary tract. Take 30–50 drops of pilosella tincture in a little water 3 times a day before meals.

- Cranberry: Cranberry is a diuretic well known for its disinfectant effect on the urinary tract. Take 20–40 drops with a little water 3 times a day before meals. (Cranberry juice is also an effective diuretic and anti-infective.)

- Couch grass: Couch grass is an excellent cleansing plant. Its preferred use is in tablet form because of its flavor. Take 1–3 tablets with a little water 3 times a day just before meals.

- Ash: A good eliminator of acids, ash, when taken in large doses, has a purgative effect. Take 1–3 tablets with a little water 3 times a day just before meals.

Some additional plant medicines and methods of preparation include:

- Goldenrod, ash, and parietaria (pellitory): For each plant mix 1–2 tablespoons per cup water. Steep for 10 minutes. Drink 3 cups daily.
- Black currant, corn silk, couch grass, elder, licorice, orthosiphon (cat's whisker), thistle: For each plant mix 1–2 tablespoons per cup water. Boil for 2 minutes, then steep 10 minutes. Drink 3 cups daily.

There are numerous commercial blends of diuretic plants available as tisanes, tinctures, tablets, and so on. These preparations are generally very effective and provide great benefit to the user.

Whey Treatment for Draining Acids

Whey is the liquid obtained from the coagulation of milk. It is released when curds are strained. The detoxifying qualities of whey have been known since antiquity. Its diuretic properties are what interest us here.

Whey owes its powerful diuretic effect to its high potassium content. By forcing excess salt out of the body, potassium prompts the elimination of fluids retained because of the presence of sodium—fluids that contain, among other things, acids. The large quantities of whey that are ingested during the course of this treatment—up to two to three quarts a day—cause the kidneys to work more intensively. The great English doctor Thomas Sydenham (1624–1689) specifically—and successfully—recommended whey as a treatment for gout, an illness caused by excess acid, particularly uric acid.

The benefits of whey for restoring the body's optimum acid–alkaline balance go beyond its ability to stimulate elimination. It is also rich in minerals (around 5 percent of its dried weight), primarily alkaline minerals such as potassium, calcium, and magnesium, which all contribute to addressing alkaline deficiencies.

Whey's alkalizing property is effective only when the whey is fresh, because whey acidifies very quickly. Even a few hours following its manufacture, whey can lose its alkaline properties. This was a very common problem in the past when treatments used only liquid whey. Today whey is available in powdered form; the powdering process arrests acidification. Sold in health food stores, it is also flavored with natural fruit extracts. The whey is reconstituted by mixing it with water according to the manufacturer's instructions. Once it has been reconstituted the liquid should be drunk quickly (within an hour), before it becomes acidic.

During the treatment, drink from three to five glasses to two to three pints of whey a day.

It is necessary, however, to give the body time to adapt. On the first day of the treatment drink only one eight-ounce glass of whey; on the second day, two glasses; and so on until you reach five glasses per day. That amount is maintained for the remainder of the treatment, which normally lasts between two and three weeks. (For those who are interested, I have written extensively on this therapy in my *La cure de petit-lait,* Geneva: Jouvence, 1994.)

ACID DRAINAGE THROUGH THE SKIN

Just like the kidneys, the sweat glands allow strong acids to be removed from the body. There are between 140 and 240 of these glands per square inch of skin, which adds up to around 2 million of these glands in the body.

The sweat glands filter out acids and toxins carried by the blood, sending them toward the body's surface, diluted in water (sweat). The blood that carries these waste products circulates in extremely fine vessels, the capillaries. Consequently, perspiration can only be abundant if there is good subcutaneous blood circulation. This can be encouraged by physical exercise, saunas, and hot baths. The muscular contractions of physical activity stimulate blood circulation, while heat causes the capillaries to dilate and also accelerates the speed with which the blood circulates.

Under normal circumstances the skin secretes between one and one and a half quarts of sweat a day. We are normally not aware of this, as the sweat evaporates immediately. Sedentary people may sweat as little as a pint a day. Elimination of acids through the skin in this case is minimal.

When stimulated by intense exercise, the skin can eliminate a pint of sweat in one hour, and considerably more if the exercise is followed by a sauna. An hour in a sauna can discharge one to one and a half quarts of sweat.

An individual suffering from a high fever eliminates similar quantities, if not more, of sweat.

Hyperthermal Baths

Insufficient elimination of acids through the skin can be corrected by physical exercise and saunas. A less well-known method is hot baths, or hyperthermal therapy. All that is required is a bathtub and hot water. The heat causes an artificial fever, which in turn stimulates a large amount of perspiration, and therefore a significant elimination of acids. Hyperthermal baths have a retraining effect on the skin. If you have poor perspiration you will, as a rule, perspire more freely after several baths.

Get into the bath when the water is at a temperature of 98.6° Fahrenheit (37° Celsius), or body tempeature, then raise the water temperature gradually by adding hot water just up to your comfort threshold. Do not bring the water to the hottest temperature you can endure; it should not be so hot that you are uncomfortable. You should be able to remain in the bath for a good quarter hour. Depending on your tolerance for heat, the temperature of the bath will be between 102° and 108° Fahrenheit (between 39° and 42° Celsius), or sometimes higher.

The purpose of this hyperthermal bath is to envelop the body in high heat. If you cannot tolerate high temperatures at all, you can still benefit by spending a longer time in the tub with the water at a comfortable temperature.

It is crucial that you allow the body to get used to the hot baths gradually, increasing the temperature and lengthening the time spent in the tub in small increments over a period of several weeks, before reaching your comfort limits.

It is not advisable to get right into a steaming hot bath even after you have built up a good tolerance. When confronted by this sudden thermal assault, the body's defenses close the pores of the skin. They are then very slow to reopen, sabotaging the purpose of the bath. So warm the bath up slowly after you get in.

When the bath is done, wrap yourself in a towel and a blanket and rest for half an hour to allow the body to finish perspiring and recover its equilibrium.

Depending on your level of vitality you can take such a bath every day for a period of two to three weeks, or every other day for several months. It is best to schedule the bath for the evening hours because it relaxes the body and encourages sound sleep.

When the body is bathed in hot water, its own internal temperature rapidly increases. This can be easily verified by taking a reading with an oral thermometer. As stated earlier, the hyperthermal bath creates an artificial fever that has the same characteristics as a genuine, natural fever.

Fever is a means of defense the body uses during illness to intensify metabolic process and accelerate the burning-off of waste products—acids among others—that saturate the body's internal environment, as well as making that environment inhospitable to the survival and reproduction of pathogens (bacteria and viruses). It is therefore a beneficial reaction that allows the body to rapidly bring its condition back to normal.

When the combustion of waste products is intensified during a fever, they are degraded and distributed throughout the body to furnish fuel for energy or cell-building material. This includes combustion of the noncirculating toxins that are deeply embedded in the body's tissues.

If you implement hyperthermal therapy too quickly you can unleash a massive discharge of deeply embedded toxins, causing what is known as a cleansing crisis. When the embedded toxins are brought suddenly to the circulatory level and added to the toxins already in circulation, the ability of the organs of elimination to oxidize and get rid of them can easily be overwhelmed. Some very unpleasant symptoms, such as headaches, nausea, and rheumatic-like crises, can result. These can be avoided by starting the therapy gradually and by draining the acids in circulation before starting an intensive hyperthermal treatment.

Drinking a sweat-stimulating tisane before and after the bath is also useful. During the bath, the skin's eliminatory work can be enhanced by scrubbing or massage.

Using Medicinal Plants for Eliminating Acids Through the Skin

Medicinal plants that increase the secretion of sweat can also increase the quantity of acids eliminated from the body. Usually, however, the increased perspiration is noticeable only when the body has a reason to sweat, such as in the case of heat or physical exertion. Nevertheless, by regularly taking sweat-stimulating substances you can help your clogged pores clean themselves and work more actively.

These preparations should be taken three times daily, and the infusions should be well heated. The effect of hyperthermal baths, sweating sessions in the sauna, and physical exercise is reinforced by drinking one to two piping hot cups of a tea brewed from sweat-stimulating herbs before and after a session.

Here are several examples of medicinal plants that have sweat-stimulating properties.

MEDICINAL PLANTS FOR ELIMINATING ACIDS
THROUGH THE SKIN

- Elder: The flowers of the elder are sweat-stimulating and diuretic, and they make a very pleasant and flavorful drink. Mix 1 tablespoon of flowers per cup of hot water as an infusion. Steep for 10 minutes. Drink 3 cups daily.

- Linden: A highly popular plant, linden has long been used for its sweat-stimulating and sedative properties. Prepare as an infusion by mixing 1 heaping handful of flowers per cup of hot water, or $^1/_2$ to 1 oz (15–30 g) per quart. Steep for 10 minutes. Drink 3 or more cups daily.
- Burdock: This plant, a diuretic, promotes bile production; it is also a laxative. Burdock is often recommended as a treatment for skin disorders. Prepare as a decoction by mixing $1^1/_2$ oz (40 g) of root per quart of water. Boil for 10 minutes. Drink 3 or more cups per day. Or take 40 drops with water 3 times a day before meals.
- Wild pansy: This plant is very effective in treating skin disorders. In addition to its sweat-stimulating qualities, it is a good overall purifier. Take 20–50 drops with water 3 times a day before meals.

Plant medicines can also be prepared as tisanes and used for stimulating sweat. Linden, elder flowers, borage, balm, violet, meadowsweet, wild pansy, chamomile, sloe flowers, and primrose are all good for use as tisanes. Mix 1 tablespoon of plant matter per cup. Steep for 10 minutes. Drink 3 cups per day.

ACID DRAINAGE THROUGH THE LUNGS

The lungs play a dual role in the elimination of acid wastes from the body. On the one hand, they supply the tissues with oxygen so volatile acids can be oxidized. It is not enough for oxygen to fill the respiratory tract; the oxygen must be conducted into the tissues by the bloodstream so that the oxidation of acid wastes can occur there. On the other hand, acids are rejected by the respiratory tract in the form of carbon dioxide (CO_2). Produced within the tissues (and present there in liquid form), this carbon dioxide must make its way to the lungs and be expelled in sufficient quantity that the body is truly rid of it.

Since everyone breathes, you might wonder why there should be any problem eliminating acid wastes through the respiratory tract. But not everyone breathes the same way; breathing rate and air flow can vary significantly from one person to another, and in the same person at different times. A person at rest takes in a pint of air per breath, whereas an active individual takes in twice that much. At the height of a game an athlete may inhale five to six quarts every breath, ten to twelve times as much as a person at rest.

Although a pint of breath is enough for an individual at rest or asleep, it is insufficient for even a sedentary person working and eating. The greater the rate of activity or amount of food eaten, the greater need the body has of oxygen. When the body does not get enough oxygen to meet its needs, oxidation is poor, which increases the accumulation of acids. Furthermore, as the volume of air exhaled is reduced so is the quantity of carbon dioxide that is eliminated. The result is acidification of the body by weak acids.

Of course, acidification of the body is even greater when a person smokes. Tobacco smoking not only reduces the intake of oxygen, and therefore the oxidation of acids in the tissues, but by hardening the lungs it diminishes the elimination of carbon dioxide. Furthermore, by constantly stimulating the nervous system, tobacco creates a state of stress in the body, which results in the production of many acids. The more acidified the body becomes by smoking, the more tired the smoker is and the greater is his urge to smoke again. Because it lowers a person's need to smoke, alkalizing the inner environment is one of the best means of enabling a smoker to kick his habit.

A properly functioning oxidation system has beneficial effects on the body's pH. If you work seated in a poorly ventilated office for an entire afternoon you are prone to acidification. If you were to measure your urinary pH at that time it would be around 5 or 6. After you took a brisk walk outside in the fresh air, however, the pH would climb back up to 7 without your having to eat any alkaline food or take an alkaline supplement. But this is only true when the cause of acidification is a lack of oxygen.

Physical activity stimulates larger inhalations and exhalations, so any aerobic exercise (walking, jogging, riding a bicycle, gymnastics, and so on) is a great help in draining acids. Daily exercise is most effective because it facilitates the oxidation and elimination of volatile acids as they are produced. Accordingly, it is preferable to walk every day for thirty minutes in the fresh air than to take a three-hour walk on the weekend.

It is clear to see that the elimination of weak acids is much easier than that of strong acids; the latter can only be voided by the kidneys in fixed daily amounts. There is, however, no set daily limit for the elimination of weak (volatile) acid wastes, which are eliminated in proportion to the oxygenation that occurs during the day.

ARE FASTS AND MONODIETS EFFECTIVE METHODS OF DEACIDIFICATION?

Drainage treatments imposed to remedy ailments other than those due to acidification frequently include measures like fasts or diets restricted to a single food. This is because the restriction of food causes significant amounts of toxins to resurface from the deep tissues, whereupon they can be conducted into the organs of elimination.

These fasts or diets are not the most beneficial treatments for detoxifying the body of acid wastes, however, and therefore cannot generally be recommended. The massive influx of acids they unleash can cause hardships for individuals who suffer from an inability to metabolize acids properly.

Of all the acids that resurface from the deep tissues during a fast, only a small quantity can be eliminated in that form by the organs of elimination. All the others must either be oxidized or buffered. People who have trouble metabolizing acids even at the best of times have little chance of greater success while they fast and these acid wastes appear in greater quantities.

Buffering acids is also problematic. For one reason, the alkaline reserves are generally already depleted; for another, the person on a fast is not ingesting alkaline substances that can support the buffer system. The body therefore must withdraw more alkalines from its reserves without being able to replenish them. This can result in serious mineral depletion.

The situation is different for those who do not have any trouble metabolizing acids. During a fast, their bodies are freed of the necessity of oxidizing acids introduced into the body by food and are able to concentrate on acids already present in the tissues. Because they have a normal capacity to burn off weak acid wastes they are able to oxidize a good amount; and because they have large alkaline reserves, it is just as easy to buffer acids.

With regard to monodiets, several scenarios are possible. As a rule, monodiets are not beneficial unless they are composed of alkaline foods such as carrots or potatoes, whether the individual has trouble metabolizing acids or not. When a monodiet involves a significant intake of alkaline substances that are not accompanied by acids, these alkaline elements can be fully used to buffer the built-up acid wastes. Furthermore, the energy saved on the digestive level by not having to deal with complicated meals can be utilized to intensify the elimination of acids by the kidneys and sweat glands.

Monodiets composed of acidifying foods, in contrast, are distinctly harmful, because the intake of these foods is not compensated for by alkaline foods. To neutralize these acids—both those that are already built up in the body and those introduced by the monodiet—the body is forced to withdraw what it needs entirely from its reserves without being able to replenish them through new food intake.

Monodiets composed of acid foods—like fruits—are to be strictly avoided by individuals who have trouble metabolizing acids, but are strongly recommended for others because of their ability to oxidize acids. These foods are transformed into alkaline substance that help alkalize their body's internal environment.

8

Alkaline Energy Boosters

In addition to taking alkaline supplements to support the body's removal of acid wastes, you may also wish to try energy boosters rich in vitamins and minerals to increase your overall vitality. The most common products of this nature are bee pollen, wheat germ, and brewer's yeast. These products and other energy boosters contain a wide range of nutrients in their natural state, which are very easy for the body to assimilate and represent a sure source of revitalization.

Unfortunately, a number of these products are acidifying and therefore not recommended if you are suffering from any of the disorders due to acidification. Among these is sea buckthorn, which is rich in vitamin C and silica; brewer's yeast, which contains purines, the precursors to uric acid; and bee pollen and, to a lesser extent, royal jelly. It may not be necessary to avoid such products completely, but their use is a delicate matter. It is preferable to use alkaline energy boosters, which include spirulina, blackstrap molasses, ginseng, wheat germ, and halibut liver oil.

The properties, indications, and instructions for using

these energy boosters are detailed below. There is no reason whatsoever that you cannot use a supplement and an energy booster at the same time. There is no risk of overdose or an ineffective double application, because the energy boosters are not characterized by their high mineral content but by their high content of vitamins, trace elements, and other nutrients.

Spirulina

Spirulina is an algae that grows in fresh water. It thrives best in alkaline waters with a pH that falls anywhere between 8.5 and 11. The use of spirulina as a food is not of recent origin. Traditionally, various African peoples have eaten it to vary their diet (which is essentially composed of millet). The Aztecs cultivated this algae in their lakes during an earlier era. Harvested with the help of fine mesh baskets that let the water run out but retained the "green foam," the foam was set out to dry, then transported throughout the Aztec empire.

The subject of numerous studies, spirulina is recognized today as an energy booster of the first order. It contains more protein, more beta-carotene (vitamin A), vitamin B_{12}, iron, and gamma-linolenic acid (vitamin F) than any other food known. Its vitamin E content is equal to that of wheat germ, otherwise its most abundant source. Spirulina's concentration of calcium and magnesium is equivalent to that of milk. Furthermore, it contains a complete range of vitamins, minerals, and trace elements.

A third of an ounce (10 g) of spirulina powder is enough to cover the daily need for vitamin B_{12} five times over, four times that for vitamin A, 83 percent of the daily requirement for iron, 30 percent of vitamin B_2, and 25 percent of vitamin B_1.

Spirulina is particularly recommended for fatigue, anemia, eyesight problems, menstrual problems, and skin disorders. In addition, it helps strengthen the immune system and facilitates the elimination of toxins that have collected inside the body.

It comes in the form of a deep-green powder with a faint aroma and also in tablets or capsules.

When combined with foods, spirulina turns them all green. For this reason it is most often used in tablet or capsule form for therapies intended to boost the body's vitality. A tablet generally contains 500 mg of spirulina. The recommended daily dosage for intensive treatments is $1/3$ ounce (10 g), which corresponds to 20 tablets, or a heaping tablespoon of powder. For maintenance therapies or when there are no urgent health issues, the doses can easily be divided into halves or thirds. Spirulina tablets should be taken with water three times a day before meals; the powder is usually eaten in combination with food.

Blackstrap Molasses

Blackstrap molasses is a byproduct of the pressing of sugar cane. It is a sugar-rich sap that has a high content of minerals, vitamins, and trace elements.

To separate the sugar from the rest of the elements, the sap is heated in a vat. The heat causes the sugar to crystallize; the crystals sink to the bottom of the vat and are harvested as whole or natural sugar. What remains on the top is a thick syrup containing the essential nutrients of the sugar cane.

Thus, whole sugar obtained through this process is not as whole as it could be. In fact, true whole sugar contains blackstrap molasses and sugar. It is produced without cooking by exposing sugar cane sap to the sun in large flat tubs so the liquid content evaporates.

Although it still contains sugar, blackstrap molasses is primarily used for its high mineral content. Three and a half ounces (100 g) of blackstrap molasses contains 1,900 to 3,300 mg of potassium, 800 to 1,400 mg of calcium, 300 to 400 mg of magnesium, 15 to 28 mg of iron, and so on. Its potassium content is higher, gram for gram, than that of soy, brewer's yeast, vegetables, or fruits, all foods considered the most important sources of potassium.

Blackstrap molasses is as rich in magnesium as wheat germ, almonds, figs, and dates, which are all generally recommended as sources of this important mineral. Likewise, iron is present in higher levels in blackstrap molasses than in liver, spinach, apricots, or eggs.

Blackstrap molasses is especially recommended for anemia, cramps, edema, rheumatism, insomnia, and stress.

It is available in liquid or solid (flake) form. It has a slightly sugary flavor with a pronounced taste of sugar cane.

The daily dose is 2 to 3 full teaspoons of liquid, or 1 to 2 tablespoons of the flakes. It can be eaten at one time or divided into three daily doses in the form of a hot or cold drink. For a hot beverage, the blackstrap molasses is blended directly with water; for a cold drink, it must first be dissolved in hot water before cold water is added.

It is advisable to drink this mixture slowly and hold it in the mouth long enough to mix it with a good amount of saliva in order to avoid bloating and flatulence.

Blackstrap molasses treatments generally last one to two months, but can be extended if necessary.

Ginseng

Ginseng is a plant native to the Far East that grows in the underbrush of woods and forests. It has been recognized and used for more than four thousand years for its curative and energy-boosting properties. At one time it was so esteemed it cost its own weight in gold.

The root is the part of the plant that is utilized. Over the course of its growth the root acquires enormous proportions in comparison with the root-to-stem proportion of most other plants. The ginseng root can grow to four feet in length and four inches in width, whereas the stem reaches a height of only twelve to thirty-two inches. The root must be at least six or seven years old before it is harvested. The wealth of ginseng's properties can be gauged from the exhaustion of the soil it grows in: after harvest, the ground must be left fallow for twelve years before it can again be used.

Ginseng root is characterized primarily by its high content of B vitamins, but it also contains vitamins A, C, D, and E, as well as an assortment of minerals and trace elements. Its healing properties appear to derive from a substance called ginsenoid. Preparations with a ginseng base should contain at least 6 percent of this substance.

There are many uses for ginseng, among them treating states of exhaustion and chronic fatigue, degenerative illnesses, depression, nervous system disorders, diabetes, and stress, as well as problems with liver function, memory, and convalescence.

In the past, ginseng treatments simply consisted of eating a small piece of the root on a daily basis. Today, liquid ginseng extract is the preferred method of use because it provides a concentrated form of the plant's active principles. The dosage level should be specified by the extract's manufacturer. Usually the extract comes with a small spoon made to hold the recommended dosage.

Treatments can extend from four to six weeks, and can be repeated as needed over the year.

Wheat Germ Sprouts

The germ is the most nutritious part of the wheat seed. The germ contains in concentrated form the major portion of the nutrients necessary for the plant's future growth: amino acids, essential fatty acids, numerous minerals, trace elements, all the B vitamins, and a high concentration of vitamin E. This exceptional nutrient content is what permits the plant to grow so explosively during its first days of life.

Surprisingly, the growth of the germ does not reduce its reserves but increases them. This makes the wheat germ even richer than it was before germination. Thanks to enzymes, new nutrients are produced. For $3^{1}/_{2}$ ounces (100 g) of wheat germ sprouts, the level of calcium rises from 45 to 71 mg, and that of magnesium from 133 to 342 mg. Vitamin content increases 20 percent for vitamin B_1, 45 percent for vitamin B_5, 200 percent for vitamin B_6, 225 percent for the proto-vitamin A, 300 percent for vitamin E, and 500 percent for vitamin C.

To sprout wheat, place the grains in a glass of water for twelve hours, then spread them on a plate near a window (for the light) and moisten them twice a day. Within three or four days the germ will sprout. It first appears as a white tip, then lengthens into a short stem that gradually changes color from white to green.

Wheat germ sprouts can be eaten when the sprout has reached a length of $^{1}/_{10}$ to $^{1}/_{5}$ inch (3 to 5 mm). At this stage it is still white. The germ is eaten with the grain and the tiny roots that have formed. It has a pleasant flavor and is an especially good addition to salads.

To have a daily supply of germinated wheat sprouts, start a new batch every day on a plate. Sprout trays with several levels are available commercially; they can replace plates and are much more convenient to use.

In addition to its energy-boosting properties, wheat germ is indicated for hypotension, depression, a tendency toward thrombosis (blood clots), and painful or irregular menstrual periods.

The daily dose is a level tablespoon of dried wheat seeds. Because of the sprouts' extremely revitalizing properties, an overdose can lead to a state of physical or psychic excitation. Sprouted wheat germ is therefore not recommended for those with high blood pressure, and its consumption in the evening is not advised. The daily dose can be taken at one time, either with breakfast or lunch.

The treatment generally lasts two to three weeks, and can be repeated as needed.

Halibut Liver Oil

Halibut is a fish found in the waters of the North Atlantic whose liver contains an oil that is quite rich in vitamin D. It contains 2 to 3 million international units (IU) of vitamin D per $3^1/_2$ ounces (100 g), whereas the other foods with the highest vitamin D content—butter, eggs, and cheese—have only 200 IU per 7 ounces (200 g).

Vitamin D not only encourages the absorption of calcium on the intestinal level, but it also contributes to maintaining a constant level of blood calcium, which allows the cells access to calcium at all times. Vitamin D also promotes the ability of calcium to remain fixed to the skeletal structure, therefore conferring solidity to the bones. Both the bloodstream and the skeleton are two important reserves from which the body can withdraw calcium in its fight against acidification.

Halibut liver oil is especially recommended for people suffering from acidification, because it prevents the decalcification of the skeleton due to acidity, as well as that caused by a deficiency in vitamin D.

In addition to vitamin D, halibut liver oil contains large quantities of vitamin A, whose well-known role in the optimal health of the eyes and skin is supplemented by its action on the skeleton. As a co-factor of vitamin D, vitamin A contributes to the formation of bones and to calcium retention.

Halibut liver oil is generally recommended during the winter, because this is the season that receives the least sunlight. The sun plays a significant role in the calcification of the skeleton, as the skin can manufacture vitamin D when it is exposed to sunlight.

This oil can treat rickets, decalcification problems, bone fractures, osteoporosis, and a tendency to dental cavities. It is also recommended for the growing years and for menopause.

Today the oil is sold in capsules to be swallowed with water. As vitamin D is a lipid-soluble vitamin, it is better digested and assimilated by the body if it is taken in the middle of a meal, preferably one that contains some fatty foods.

It is important to follow the manufacturer's dosage instructions, because an overdose of vitamin D can be harmful to a person's health.

These treatments can extend for two to three months.

Acidified individuals do not need to wait for winter to begin their treatment, but can start it whenever they please. Subsequently, the treatment should be repeated on a yearly basis during the cold months.

Sicknesses do not appear suddenly and for no reason; they are the result of causes that need to be dealt with in order for the sickness to disappear. The cause of acid problems in the body lies in the way people eat and live. The information in this book shows you how to modify these factors in order to be healthy again. I wish readers every success in your quest for good health.

URINARY pH RECORD

Date	Morning	Noon	Evening	Observations

Resources
⤳

ALKALINE SUPPLEMENTS

Distribution Biobasit
Exclusive U.S. and Canadian distributor for Biosana products,
   including Erbasit and Nimbasit
1053, rue Châteauneuf
Saint-Jérome Québec J5L 1H7
Tel: 450-565-1757
Toll free: 800-643-8998
biobasit@ca.inter.net

Kousmine Foundation
This company ships worldwide; manufacturers of
   Megabase, Equilibre-Vital
39, Rue de la Madeleine
1800 Vevey
Switzerland
Tel: 41-21-922-5854

pHion Nutrition
Manufactures pH test strips, alkalizing supplements
7741 E Gray Rd
Scottsdale AZ 85260
www.ph-ion.com
Toll Free: 888-744-8589

Index